# Limiting Harm in Health Care:
# A Nursing Perspective

For Grace.

# Limiting Harm in Health Care: A Nursing Perspective

Edited by

## Frank Milligan

Senior Lecturer,
University of Luton

## Kate Robinson

Deputy Vice Chancellor (Academic),
University of Luton

**Blackwell**
Science

© 2003 by Blackwell Science Ltd,
a Blackwell Publishing Company
Editorial Offices:
9600 Garsington Road, Oxford OX4 2DQ, UK
  *Tel:* +44 (0)1865 776868
Blackwell Publishing Inc., 350 Main Street,
Malden, MA 02148-5018, USA
  *Tel:* +1 781 388 8250
Iowa State Press, a Blackwell Publishing
Company, 2121 State Avenue, Ames, Iowa
50014-8300, USA
  *Tel:* +1 515 292 0140
Blackwell Publishing Asia Pty Ltd,
550 Swanston Street, Carlton South,
Victoria 3053, Australia
  *Tel:* +61 (0)3 9347 0300
Blackwell Wissenschafts Verlag,
Kurfürstendamm 57, 10707 Berlin, Germany
  *Tel:* +49 (0)30 32 79 060

First published 2003 by Blackwell Science Ltd

Library of Congress
Cataloging-in-Publication Data
Limiting harm in health care : a nursing
  perspective / edited by Frank Milligan, Kate
  Robinson.
    p. ; cm.
Includes bibliographical references and index.
  ISBN 0-632-05996-6 (hardback)
  1. Nursing errors—Prevention.
  [DNLM: 1. Medical Errors—prevention &
  control.   2. Accident Prevention.   3. Nursing
  Care—standards.   4. Quality Assurance,
  Health Care.   WB 100 L734 2003]   I. Milligan,
  Frank.   II. Robinson, Kate.

RT85.6 .L54 2003
362.1′73′068—dc21
                                    2002154162

ISBN 0-632-05996-6

A catalogue record for this title is available from
the British Library

Set in 10.5/12.5pt Palatino
by DP Photosetting, Aylesbury, Bucks
Printed and bound in Great Britain by
MPG Books Ltd, Bodmin, Cornwall

For further information on
Blackwell Publishing, visit our website:
www.blackwellpublishing.com

The opinions expressed in this book are those of the editors and authors concerned. These views are not
necessarily those held by Blackwell Publishing.

# Contents

v

Contents

Contents

Contents

viii

Contents

# *Preface*

This book is for all those working in health care who seek to enhance their practice by reducing levels of unnecessary harm caused to users of the various health services. It will be of particular interest to nurses but most of the issues analysed are of relevance to a wider audience including those who use the health service. The origins of the book lie in our own experiences. Between us we have worked in a wide range of health care environments across both clinical and educational settings and it is that background which informed the need for this text. Although the book is British in emphasis, much of what is discussed here will be relevant to other countries in which a western medical approach dominates health care. In putting together the team of authors we have tried to include a range of different environments and issues. However, what we hope the team has in common is a critical rather than a complacent view of the benefits of health care.

The editors hope to engage the reader in a more critical view of practice. By critical we mean a perspective that seeks to acknowledge both strengths and weaknesses in health care. An increase in intervention inevitably brings an increase in risk and some aspects of health care bring with them significant risks of unnecessary harm. We were particularly keen to acknowledge that as the scope of nursing practice expands, so does the possibility of causing harm. We hope that this book, and the range of examples included, will encourage practitioners to examine critically current practice and the possibilities of unnecessary harm inherent in it. Efforts to reduce such harm offer the opportunity significantly to enhance health care.

# Contributors

Angeline Burke is Senior Policy Officer at the Association of Community Health Councils for England and Wales (ACHCEW). (Community Health Councils are independent bodies established to represent the interests of the public in the NHS. The ACHCEW represents these interests at a national level.) Her work includes writing policy and research papers such as the influential *Hungry in Hospital?* which looked at malnutrition in hospitals from the patient's perspective. She is responsible for managing the Association's annual nationwide Casualty Watch, an independent survey of waiting times in Accident and Emergency (A&E) departments.

Marilyn Burn is an RN with a degree in Health Care who works as a sister on the Coronary Care Unit at Bedford Hospital. Her clinical work has been within the field of coronary care nursing. An interest in multidisciplinary work has led to her lecturing on aspects of clinical audit in cardiology. She has been one of the team involved in ensuring the National Service Framework targets are met within the local acute Trust setting.

Uttom Chowdhury qualified in medicine at Manchester University Medical School. After working as a psychiatrist for several years and obtaining Membership of the Royal College of Psychiatrists, he went on to specialise in child psychiatry. He trained as a specialist registrar on the Great Ormond Street Hospital Child Psychiatry scheme. He currently works as a Consultant in Child and Adolescent Psychiatry for Bedfordshire and Luton Community NHS Trust. His particular interests include neurodevelopmental disorders including Attention Deficit Hyperactivity Disorder, autism and Tourette's syndrome. His other research interests include neuroimaging, anorexia nervosa and obsessive compulsive disorder in children.

Denise Flisher is an RN working as a Cardiac Services Manager at Bedford Hospital. Her clinical background includes being senior sister on a coronary care unit and she has also worked as a resuscitation training officer. More recently she has been actively involved in the implementation of the National Service Framework for Coronary Heart Disease at regional level. She is currently undertaking a Masters Degree in Professional Practice and has had several articles published on resuscitation and thrombolysis. She has recently led the development of the specialist nurse roles of 'heart failure' and 'rapid access' nurse.

Ponnusamy Ganeson, BSc (Hons) qualified as a Registered Nurse (mental health) in 1986. He worked in acute psychiatry before focusing on work in child and adolescent mental health (CAMH). He qualified as a Family Therapist with the Institute of Family Therapy, London and is a trained facilitator in Webster-Stratton parent training. He has pioneered the use of group work in social skills and loss issues for children and adolescents and is currently working as a Lead Clinician in Community Mental Health Nursing for CAMH service for the Bedfordshire and Luton NHS Community Trust. He lectures part time in counselling and is actively involved in delivering a CAMH teaching programme to primary care workers. His other area of interest is cognitive behaviour therapy.

Jennifer Kelly qualified as an RN in 1980 at Addenbrooke's hospital in Cambridge. She has worked in a variety of clinical areas including oncology, A&E, surgery and as a tissue viability nurse. A long-standing interest in nurse education resulted in her qualifying and working first as a clinical teacher and then as a nurse tutor. She has a Masters degree in biochemical pharmacology and has published a number of papers and a book on pharmacology in relation to nursing. Recently she has developed a module in Medicines Management and has become involved in the degree level drug prescribing course.

Joan P. McDowall is a graduate of Loughborough University who holds both a nursing and a midwifery qualification. After working in clinical practice as a midwife she held several posts at different levels of management including at national level. Joan has also worked as an industrial relations officer and as a Senior Midwifery Adviser/Senior Professional Officer with the Royal College of Midwives. She has recently retired as a Senior Lecturer from the

University of Luton where she was involved in pre and post registration nurse education.

Alastair McElroy is a Registered Mental Nurse and works as a Principal Lecturer in Mental Health at the University of Luton. His professional and academic interests have increasingly focused on the management of individuals with personality disorders. This was reflected in his PhD thesis, which explored the psychological care mental health nurses offered to self-harming patients. He continues to work with staff and patients in order to develop and evaluate the care offered to this group based on the outcomes of the study.

Frank Milligan is an RN who works as a Senior Lecturer at the University of Luton. His clinical experience includes areas such as orthopaedics, intensive care and haematology nursing. More recently he has acted as the educational link to wards for acute care of the elderly. His educational experience includes both pre and post registration nursing programmes and a number of curriculum developments. He has published on a range of educational and clinical issues.

Donald Richardson was a general practitioner for 32 years. For most of that time he was involved in medical politics. He was an elected member and Chairman of a Local Medical Committee, representing the views of GPs to the NHS, a member and Vice Chairman of an Area Health Authority and a Regional Health Authority for ten years. After retiring he spent six years as the full-time Secretary of three Local Medical Committees. He was a general practice adviser for the National Sick Doctor Scheme, instrumental in establishing research to assess the scope and benefits of counselling support for GPs and helped to set up the local procedures to deal with poor performance as required by the GMC. He still assists practitioners as a Clinical Complaints Adviser for the Medical Defence Union. More recently, he has been Medical Director of a site of NHS Direct and Medical Adviser to an ambulance service.

Kate Robinson is currently working as the Deputy Vice Chancellor (Academic) the University of Luton. She is qualified as a Nurse and a Health Visitor and holds degrees in History and Health Studies. She has lectured and published in the areas of client–practitioner interaction, including mediated interaction, and equalities issues.

Stuart Thompson is an RN with a BA in Healthcare. He is the Education Facilitator for Bedfordshire and Hertfordshire NHS Direct. His clinical background includes experience in general surgery, orthopaedics, gastrointestinal and colorectal surgery. Stuart has worked within telephone triage since 1999, and is responsible for developing links with clinical areas and providing teaching and education support for NHS Direct staff. Stuart is also a member of the NHS Direct National Training Team, which is responsible for the implementation of the New Clinical Assessment System, the computer decision support software for NHS Direct.

John Wilkinson trained as an RN in London and has worked clinically in psychiatric, adult and critical care settings. He has a degree in psychology and a higher degree in nursing and has held posts in higher education where he has worked as a lecturer and manager. John returned to the NHS and was an assistant clinical director for education, research and practice development in an acute trust prior to taking up his present position as an Officer with the Royal College of Nursing, Eastern Region.

Richard Winter is an RN who is currently Clinical Director Nursing and acting General Manager for NHS Direct Bedfordshire and Hertfordshire. He has worked in the health service for 15 years in a variety of roles and has a particular interest in change management, having implemented nursing information systems in an acute trust. More recently he has been a national clinical lead for the Clinical Assessment System (CAS) Training Team and has been the nurse lead for the National Interactive Web Based Triage/health information project team.

Valerie Young is an RN in both the general and mental health fields. She also holds a BA (Hons) Sociology and a Higher Diploma in Health Visiting. She works as a Senior Teaching Fellow at the University of Luton in the Faculty of Health and Social Science, teaching on palliative care, reflective practice and clinical supervision courses.

# Acknowledgements

The editors would like to thank all the contributors to this book for the time and effort that they have given to this project. We would also like to thank Cheryl Watson, Penny Fasey and Donald Richardson for their comments on the manuscript, Mary Hahn for proof reading and Nigel Ingram and Alan Dickinson for their advice on aspects of Chapter 13. We would also like to acknowledge the contribution made by Garry Ashwell and the other learning resource staff at the University of Luton for their help with obtaining materials and referencing, and Martina Brennan for her support and patience.

A special thank you goes to Beth Knight at Blackwell Publishing for her help throughout preparation and completion of the book, and finally to Josette who had to live with the idea and project for the best part of two years.

## Editors' note

It is acknowledged that individual authors will not necessarily agree with all the points put forward in chapters other than their own. However, all the contributors hold the common goal of reducing unnecessary harm in health care.

# 1. *Introduction, Aims and Mapping Health Care*

*Frank Milligan and Kate Robinson*

> 'Those who claim authority to name problems in the human world must be prepared to understand themselves as part of the problem structure they have created'
>
> Fenwick and Parsons, 1998 p. 64

## Introduction

The central idea on which this book is based is a simple one. It is that there is a significant amount of unnecessary harm done to people within the current medically dominated health care systems, and as nurse roles continue to expand, so the amount of harm nurses are causing may increase. But this is not an instructional text about how to manage risk; rather it is a book which attempts to look at the issues in some new ways and in different contexts.

The term *iatrogenesis* is surprisingly little used in health care and may therefore be unfamiliar to many health care practitioners, but it is important to them and to us because it means 'doctor generated harm' (Illich, 1990). It refers to the unnecessary harm that occurs as a consequence of the dominance of a particular system of health care provision, one in which medical definitions and medical power prevail. The harm is 'unnecessary' in the sense that it is a by-product of particular methods of health care which may involve a degree of injury, dependence, discomfort and pain. While some of this may be inevitable – injections often hurt, however careful the practitioner – some could be avoided either through more careful (in the literal sense) practice or by a reconsideration of the relevance and necessity of some kinds of practice. The challenge, for everyone working in health care, is to consider how individual practice may be contributing to medical harm, and how they are contributing to

1

or resisting the systems which result in harm. This is an important time to ask these questions for two reasons. First, there is an increasing awareness amongst the public that health care may be harmful, resulting in increasing questioning of health care practitioners. Secondly, the way in which roles and responsibilities are being assigned between health care workers means that many will be working in unfamiliar territory and will be moving outside their 'taken for granted' competence.

The system of health care to which the arguments in this book are mainly addressed is that which was developed largely in western Europe and the USA, and which now has a predominate position throughout the world. It is based on the knowledge developed by the bio-sciences and has largely neglected the knowledge base of traditional healers. The predominate locus of power in this health care system has been the medical profession, but this is being increasingly challenged both by the state and the public, on the grounds that they want to know what they are paying for, and by other practitioners in other health care occupations who, for a number of reasons, want 'a larger slice of the action'. This book brings together a range of different points of view and experiences in order to begin to explore how things might be different in the future. It contends that the influence and actions of western medicine are at times a threat to health, the significance of which is frequently forgotten within medically influenced health care systems, and that all of us who work within the system should reflect on ways in which our strategies for helping ourselves, our professional group and our patients reduce or increase the risk of harm.

It may seem paradoxical to talk of medical harm, after all, the aim of medicine, as stipulated in the Hippocratic oath, is to do no harm (Sharpe & Faden, 1998). However, as the next chapter will demonstrate, unnecessary harm can and does occur. The UK public is now familiar with cases like that of Dr Shipman and the Bristol Royal Infirmary Inquiry. The former was a general practitioner (GP) convicted of the murder of 15 of his elderly female patients (Baker, 2000). It appears that his status as a doctor shielded him from the kind of enquiries which might have stopped him much sooner. It is true that the patients of GPs die, but not normally in the numbers and with the characteristics with which his patients died. But questions were not asked and he continued in practice (Whittle & Ritchie, 2000). The Bristol Royal Infirmary Inquiry (2001) was initiated after it became clear that mortality rates in children undergoing heart surgery at this centre were unusually high. It concluded that a 'club culture' existed, where too much power lay in the hands of too few people, and about one-third of all children undergoing surgery received less than adequate care. The findings and recommendations made in the Bristol Inquiry were, with a few exceptions, accepted by the Government in its response to the report (DoH, 2002). These events may be extreme examples, but they show how systems and statuses in health care that are taken for granted can eventually lead to a position in which public trust is shattered.

## The aims of this book

We would suggest that all those contributing to health care might usefully ask themselves, 'what might I be doing that is potentially iatrogenic?' With these issues in mind, the authors of this book wish to:

i.   question our faith in the effectiveness of western medicine and its contribution to health care
ii.  clarify the nature and extent of iatrogenic harm
iii. explore the expanding scope of nursing practice and relate this to issues raised through the concept of iatrogenic harm
iv.  give clear examples of the negative effects of the current medical approach to certain health issues
v.   explore the implications of the issues raised for future health care practice and offer suggestions on ways of reducing unnecessary harm.

This chapter now moves on to a brief description of the historically close relationship between medicine and nursing. It is suggested that any substantial attempt to understand the potential contribution of nursing to health care must first acknowledge the limits of western medicine. An analogy is drawn between maps of the world and a hypothetical map of health care to help us step back from our taken for granted assumptions. Some examples of the problems created by medicine are given, before the repercussions of these issues on the expanding scope of nursing practice are briefly reviewed.

## Doctors and nurses

Doctors and nurses in western societies have developed a close working relationship since the early nineteenth century. It is a relationship that carries a high profile in popular culture, being the subject of everything from children's games through to romantic fiction (Williams, 2000). Doctors are commonly associated with treatment and cure, whilst nurses are linked to care and the everyday chores of supporting those unable too fully aid themselves (Davies, 1995). As with so much of modern life, this relationship is as subject to change as the tasks that both disciplines are expected and obliged to perform. However, various problems with the relationship, not least in terms of gender and status, have been and continue to be explored (for example Gamarnikow, 1978; Mackay, 1993; Williams, 2000).

Although some of the tasks may change, for example who takes a blood pressure reading or who prescribes a pain relieving drug, the social and gendered structures in terms of the difference in status between medicine and nursing remain somewhat static. Some suggest that the relationship is in fact wounded, being based upon nineteenth century gendered notions of master–servant subordination (Wicks, 1998). Having said this, there are increasing challenges to both the status and gender divisions between the two. For example, nursing continues to move up the academic scale and to take on wider and more complex roles in health care (Gott, 2000). Substantial shifts have also been seen in terms of the gender division between medicine and nursing and half of medical school entrants in the UK are now female (Davies *et al.*, 1999). Against this background nursing has struggled to make sense of its contribution within health care. Davies (1995), a sociologist who has published widely on nursing and health policy, has argued that nurses need to take their place in debates about public policy and health. For Davies, as for others who offer a socio-political and gendered analysis of the predicament of nursing, the voice of nursing is a disadvantaged voice.

It is suggested here that the risk for nursing staff, of actually causing and perpetuating unnecessary harm lies not just in problems created through the assimilation of new roles. Many current roles, and the context within which those roles are undertaken, actually create and perpetuate harm. What is currently seen as 'normal' (see Mackay (1993) for clarification of this word in this context) and even best practice, is leading to unacceptable levels of unnecessary harm. Because of the flawed nature of the relationship between the two occupations, which is evident through aspects of their communication with each other (Sweet & Norman, 1995), it is difficult for nurses to see and speak of the harm caused in health care.

Being clear about the roles (and potential roles) of nurses is particularly important when the boundaries between the two disciplines appear to be closing and the risk of litigation against nurses undertaking what have hitherto been medical roles, increases (Fletcher, 2000). Such analysis is particularly important as the political background can shift dramatically, as was seen in the UK following the defeat of the Conservative government in 1997. This saw a move away from the ethos of competition between the various elements within the NHS to one of collaboration and partnership (Williams, 2000). The pressures on nurses to expand the roles they undertake can therefore range from the micro level, for example pressure from their medical colleagues, to the macro context of central government initiatives.

## Seeing the limits of medicine – maps as knowledge

Being able to acknowledge the unnecessary harm and limits of medicine and medically dominated health care is a difficult task. Being an integral part of health care does not necessarily put the practitioner in a strong position for evaluating it. Much has been researched and written on the occupational socialisation processes nurses are subject to (for examples see Mackay *et al.*, 1998), and those processes have generally not encouraged such critique. Furthermore, nurses reflect the values and beliefs of the society of which they are a component, and their views on the goals and achievements of medically dominated health care reflect that. These factors create a position in which it can be difficult for nurses to be objective or critical about the limits of the systems they work within and perpetuate.

An illustration of this difficulty is offered in Fig. 1.1. It is commonly assumed that the map of the world represents the world. We believe we know which way is up and when shown a map with south at the top (see Fig. 1.1), would probably want to turn it round to make immediate sense of it. Such a view of the world is pervasive and you will rarely see any other depiction of our planet. But our planet is a globe floating in space and there is, therefore, no top or bottom. 'North at the top' was not always the convention in map making; some early navigators used south as the top of their maps. The word *orientation* comes from east being the direction of the rising sun, hence it was once common practice to put east at the top of maps (Turnbull, 1993).

No map can accurately convey the relationships between, or surface areas of, different countries. Some elements will be enhanced and others lost in the attempt to replicate the world. For

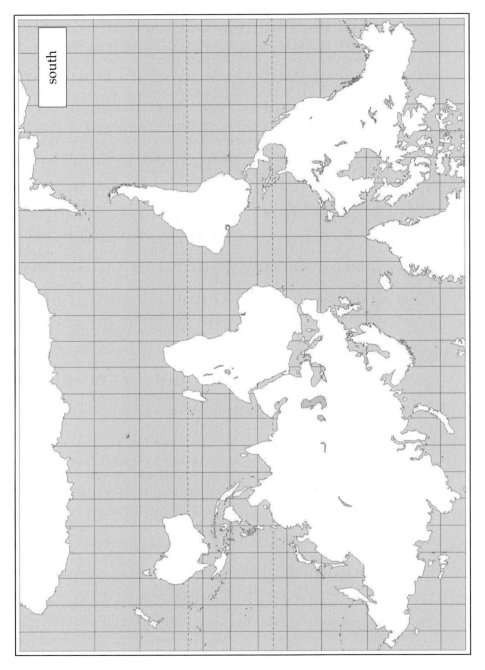

south

**Fig. 1.1** Mercator projection of the world (produced by the Cartographic Research Laboratory, University of Alabama).

example Mercator's projection, one of the commonest maps in general circulation, makes Greenland appear larger than Australia when in fact the latter is more than three times the size of Greenland (Turnbull, 1993). This effect is in part caused by giving more area to the Northern Hemisphere – the equator is not placed in the centre of the map. In this common projection of the world, Northern Hemisphere countries are 'above' others, and this implies an importance and power over those below. North became 'the top' for reasons linked to the global rise and economic dominance of northern Europe (Turnbull, 1993). Essentially a Eurocentric view was taken and early mapmakers, as inhabitants of the significant world powers of the time, predictably put themselves top-centre.

Maps are then *a* representation of the world, not *the* representation of the world. They have been used for the purposes of nationalism and Eurocentrism (Black, 1997), and '... are the product of decisions and actions taken by identifiable members of social groups in particular historical circumstances. More than a mirror of society, maps are a reciprocal part of cultural growth and influence the pattern of its development' (Hartley & Woodward, 1987 p. 506). Maps can be seen then as a metaphor for knowledge (Turnbull, 1993). Our view (gaze) of the world has been constructed through such maps. It infiltrates our perceptions and language allowing us, for example, to refer to those 'down-under'. Our gaze, our understanding of the world through north-oriented maps, is pervasive, both helpful as it allows us to discuss and move around a world we feel we understand, and limiting in that we can find other views disorientating. However, as the French writer Foucault (1991) argued, gaze is not faithful to truth nor subject to it; it dominates its masters. Although we feel we understand the globe through the maps we commonly use, that understanding is superficial and itself limiting. We are at the same time both enabled and disabled. We have come to take for granted something that is in fact a poor representation of the globe, the world upon which we live, and that representation influences our everyday thinking and understanding.

## The map of western medicine

This book is based upon the premise that our views of health and health care systems are very much like a Mercator map of the world. Consider for a moment that we have an imaginary map of modern health care. Western medicine has written itself into the top-centre (Europe) and used a wider scale for the Northern Hemisphere thereby ensuring that it looks more important than other, Southern Hemisphere, approaches to health. The equator is drawn below the centre of the map, even though the centre is a very logical place to put it. This has the effect of decreasing the importance of those therapies that are seen to be 'down under', alternative and complementary, and reduces the emphasis given to those problems medicine creates, represented in our imaginary map by Australia.

Not only is this imaginary map of health care a representation of the professional and socio-political aims of western medicine, as Mercator's projection is a representation of the socio-political aims of those that first drew it, medicine's map will also influence future health care development. It is difficult to see, when using such a map, medicine as doing anything other than good. Our view of medicine is one that interprets its success from a perspective that accentuates its success. Emphasis is rarely given to the fact that major advances in health are due to social and environmental changes (Taylor & Field, 1997), or to the unnecessary harm that western medicine and its associated systems can cause.

## *Mapping medical harm*

There are things that medicine does well. Using the biomedical model doctors have developed the means to identify and treat a significant number of health problems (Doyal, 1995). When people are taken acutely ill western medicine can offer a good deal of help, reduce suffering and sometimes save lives, and cure rates for some diseases have improved dramatically (Taylor & Field, 1997). There is however, an unjustified emphasis on acute medical care in western societies (Williams, 2000). The dramatic interventions, the emergencies, have become widely perceived as the key purpose of health care and the subject of much fiction. Examples of the latter include *Casualty*, a long-running television drama in the UK and *ER* from the USA. These, and the plethora of other similar and popular programmes, portray health care workers as lifesavers – heroes working in the face of adversity. They mirror within popular culture the western medical preference for technological intervention following a supposedly logical diagnostic process. Problems are identified and solved. They don't, however, mirror the everyday reality of health care in which acute work is but the tip of the iceberg. Beyond lies the significant burden of lay care, which takes place in people's own homes (Twigg & Aitkin, 1994). The bulk of 'carework' and 'professional care' (for clarification of these terms see Davies, 1995) take place in rehabilitation and community settings.

## *Examples of harm*

Beyond the cases of Harold Shipman and the Bristol Royal Infirmary Inquiry described in the opening of this chapter, there are other examples where some of the most apparently secure looking areas of medicine in fact raise significant problems. For example, mass screening programmes such as those for breast and cervical cancer remain controversial within the medical community. The debate includes questions about the actual impact on mortality rates, the financial cost of any health improvement gained, and the levels of error and stress caused to people subject to screening (for example Gøtzche & Olsen, 2000). These issues are discussed in more detail in Chapter 2.

In the recent debate on the length of hospital waiting lists within the NHS, it is often forgotten that unnecessary and inappropriate surgery is still commonly performed (Sharpe & Faden, 1998; Ritchie Report, 2000). For example, around 25% of appendectomies are performed on people with a normal appendix (Styrud *et al.*, 1999). Although the health risks from a ruptured appendix are significant, the risks from unnecessary anaesthetics and surgery should not be underestimated. Taking a historical perspective, it is clear that some surgery, for example the high numbers of tonsillectomies that once seemed necessary, are now rarely performed (Sharpe & Faden, 1998). No doubt, we will look back on some of the surgery we take for granted today in a similar manner.

Medicine has also helped exacerbate the current rise in antibiotic-resistant micro-organisms through the over-prescription of anti-biotics (Dutton, 1988). The rise in such organisms is now seen as a central concern for health care, even calling into question the future of the large general hospital. The National Audit Office (Comptroller and Auditor General, 1999) has released figures stating that around 5,000 people die from hospital acquired infections in the UK every year.

In the USA, the administration of President Clinton initiated investigations into levels of medical harm and estimated 98,000 people a year were dying as a direct consequence of medical intervention. An editor of this report subsequently claimed that this figure was an underestimate as it did not take into account deaths outside of the inpatient setting (Woods, 2000). This is interesting as much of the research into medical harm concentrates on the hospital setting, thereby underestimating the possible levels of harm occurring within the wider community. Recently research has been started in England to replicate the work of the classic Harvard

(Brennan *et al.*, 1991; Leape *et al.*, 1991) and Australian (Wilson *et al.*, 1995) studies into adverse events in hospitals. Adverse events are defined as unintended injuries caused by medical management rather than the disease process. The retrospective review of 1014 medical and nursing records showed that 10.8% of patients experienced adverse events of which about half were judged to be preventable (Vincent *et al.*, 2001).

Leape (1999) has brought together evidence on medical harm from a variety of studies and claimed that if the rates were typical then across the USA 180,000 deaths a year are the result of iatrogenic, medically generated injury. This, Leape points out, is the equivalent of three jumbo-jet crashes every two days. Furthermore, the scale of non-fatal errors remains largely hidden. The aviation analogy is interesting here for two reasons. First, that industry works on a 0.1% error rate, which even then is seen as too high, whereas evidence from medicine suggests that error rates are around 1% (Leape, 1999). Second, it rather neatly encapsulates the problem facing nursing as addressed in this book. We have been, in our historical role of assistants to medicine (Gamarnikow, 1978; Wicks, 1998), the equivalent of stewards/stewardesses in these imaginary aeroplanes, but we are increasingly being asked actually to fly them through the expansion of nursing roles. It is argued that the goal for nursing and others working in health care should be to help move error rates towards aviation, as opposed to medical, levels.

## Expanding nursing roles in health care

This brief sketch of unnecessary harm in health care is an introduction to the sorts of issues this book seeks to highlight. They are important because nurses are being asked to change their roles within health care (DoH, 1999a). Although this should bring with it benefits for the recipients of those services, and evidence suggests that nurses can continue to expand their contribution and make positive steps towards improving people's health status (for example Gott, 2000), it is argued that nursing needs to tread carefully on this new ground.

One of the emerging areas in which role expansion is evident is that of the nurse practitioner. In the USA, debate continues over the educational content of the preparation programmes for this role. Although these nurses have achieved a high quality, cost effective contribution to health care, some have argued that they are little more than mini doctors (Goodyear, 2000). This will be of concern to some in terms of the aims of nursing as a discrete discipline (Walsh, 2000). From the perspective of this book it is of particular concern because in taking on roles and tasks formerly undertaken by medicine, nurses may increasingly be involved in causing and/or perpetuating iatrogenic harm. As nursing roles expand, so does the risk of causing such harm. To put it simply, we may be taking over more of the work that causes unnecessary harm. The chapters that follow seek to build on these arguments and give insights into the range and diversity of unnecessary harm in health care.

## *The chapters*

In order to offer a critique on the limits of contemporary medical practice, it is necessary first to be clear on its nature and aims, and Chapter 2 addresses this task. It clarifies the approach of western medicine, including its concerns and goals, and explores the nature of iatrogenic harm. It argues that iatrogenesis is not just about the micro issues of medical harm, for example removal of the wrong kidney during surgery, but also the macro context, including our social and cultural responses to health challenges (Illich, 1990).

Chapter 3 examines the importance attached to being a professional and questions whether it offers any defence against doing harm. Although the status of nursing as a profession remains contentious (Davies, 1995), there is no doubt that medicine is seen as a profession. While such status brings with it considerable advantages for the practitioner and indeed society in general, this does not come without a price which may be paid by individuals and by society. As nursing changes its sphere of practice influence, so it might want to ponder the importance, value and consequences of pursuing professional status. Chapter 4 continues this theme through exploring the expanding boundaries of current nursing practice, and the limits, or lack of these, within which nursing operates. It clarifies the current policy in relation to the expanding scope of professional practice, statutory requirements and the guidance given to nurses on these matters. This context is critically explored and the possible repercussions, in terms of the potential risks of doing harm, are considered along with clarification of the current legal status and scope of nursing practice.

The following chapters move from general commentary on the profession to more specific examples of practice. Adverse drug reactions and mistakes made in drug prescription, calculation and administration are all known to cause a significant amount of harm in modern health care. Similarly, compliance with prescribed drug regimes is also known to be poor. These issues are debated in Chapter 5 in the context of the present moves to expand nurse prescribing in the UK. The problems sometimes caused by alternative and complementary therapy medicines are also explored. Chapter 6 examines the rise in drug use to control children's behaviour. This is an example of iatrogenic harm at the social and cultural levels, through the generation of a new diagnostic category that paves the way for medical intervention. Until recently it was very unusual for young children to be prescribed drugs that act on the central nervous system for behavioural problems, yet there have been dramatic increases in prescription rates, especially in those labelled as having hyperactivity disorders since the early 1990s. It is argued that this is a clear example of medicalisation – the labelling of a group for the purposes of justifying medical treatment – and that the treatment given is frequently inappropriate as less invasive forms of therapy could be considered.

Chapter 7 explores the limits of a medicalised approach to mental health work. A contrast is made between 'medical treatment', which remains largely reliant upon physical interventions, and 'psycho-social care' which emphasises the importance of dialogue and relationships. Implicit in the concept of mental illness is an assumption that the effects of psychological interventions are more or less innocuous because they are 'only talk', whereas 'real' treatment comes from medical doctors. However, the author contends that people can be as much harmed by words as they can be by physical interventions, and that nursing interventions can themselves be harmful.

Chapter 8 gives a lay perspective on the experiences of challenging health care practitioners through complaints procedures. The Community Health Councils have acted for many years as the advocates of people using the National Health Service (NHS) and the chapter explores a number of the issues from the lay viewpoint using specific examples. It is argued that complaints can be used to constructively assess the extent of, and generate a response to, concerns with regard to health care provision.

In Chapter 9 the relationship between the work of doctors and nurses is examined in the acute environment of coronary care units. The diagnoses and interventions undertaken are technical and acute in nature, placing particular strains on all the staff. It is demonstrated that nurses are doing much of the diagnostic work and can be more reliable in terms of following the prescribed treatment protocols than their junior medical colleagues. In addition, nurses are being asked to expand their roles into the administration of powerful anti-thrombolytic agents. These issues are explored within the context of implementing nurse led thrombolysis in an acute hospital trust. Chapter 10 examines the notion of iatrogenesis as harm caused through the use of medical language and goals in the palliative care setting. Drawing on stories from specialist palliative care practice, it shows how medically constructed discourse sometimes unconsciously, sometimes authoritatively, silences the voices of patients and disempowers potentially useful health care discourses.

The impact of information technology and challenges to the gate-keeping role of medicine are explored in Chapter 11. Nursing has been central to the development of the NHS Direct initiative in the UK; a telephone based information service, which may eventually replace general practitioners as the first point of contact with the health service by the community. It is argued that reference to a computer for guidance during assessment and treatment will become routine in most health care environments. NHS Direct is one of several initiatives that challenge the gate-keeping role of doctors.

As the scope of nursing practice continues to expand, so will the levels of risk, in terms of the quality of decision making, to which nurses are exposed. Medicine has become increasingly sensitive to the levels of risk its practitioners are subject to in this area. The process of decision making inevitably carries an element of risk, a notion acknowledged in recent government documents, such as *An Organisation with a Memory* (DoH, 2000; DoH 2001) and *Supporting Doctors, Protecting Patients* (DoH, 1999b). Chapter 12 describes lessons from personal medical experience and offers some response to issues raised elsewhere in the book. The final chapter does not attempt to summarise all the issues raised but rather revisits the concept of iatrogenesis in the light of the arguments made within the book. The significance and potential impact of iatrogenic harm on nursing practice are explored and the repercussions for health care are examined. Recent government initiatives on improving quality in the NHS and reducing the incidence of adverse events are outlined. Some suggestions are made with regard to reducing iatrogenic harm within the expanding scope of nursing practice, as well as proposals made for future research. These complement rather than summarise the suggestions for practice made in Chapters 5 to 11.

# References

Baker, R. (2000) *Harold Shipman's Clinical Practice 1974–1998.* Department of Health, London.

Black, J. (1997) *Maps and History. Constructing Images of the Past.* Yale University Press, New Haven, CT.

Brennan, T. A., Leape, L. L., Laird, N. M., Hebert, L., Localio, A. R., Lawthers, A. G., Newhouse, J. P., Weiler, P. C. & Hiatt, H. H. (1991) Incidence of adverse events and negligence in hospitalized patients. Results of the Harvard Medical Practice Study I. *New England Journal of Medicine.* **324,** 370–376.

Bristol Royal Infirmary Inquiry (2001) *Learning from Bristol. The report of the public inquiry into children's heart surgery at the Bristol Royal Infirmary, 1984–1995.* Department of Health, London.

Comptroller and Auditor General (2000) *The Management and Control of Hospital Acquired Infection in Acute NHS Trusts in England.* Department of Health, London.

Davies, C. (1995) *Gender and the Professional Predicament in Nursing.* Open University Press, Buckingham.

Davies, C., Salvage, J. & Smith, R. (1999) Doctors and nurses: changing family values? *British Medical Journal.* **319,** 463–464.

DoH (1999a) *Making a Difference; Strengthening the nursing, midwifery and health visitor contribution to health and health care.* Department of Health, London.

DoH (1999b) *Supporting Doctors, Protecting Patients.* Department of Health, London.

DoH (2000) *An Organisation with a Memory. Report of an expert group on learning from adverse events in the NHS chaired by the Chief Medical Officer.* The Stationery Office, London.

DoH (2001) *Building a Safer NHS for Patients: Implementing* An Organisation with a Memory. The Stationery Office, London.

DoH (2002) *Learning from Bristol: The Department of Health's response to the Report of the Public Inquiry into Children's Heart Surgery at the Bristol Royal infirmary 1984–1995.* The Stationery Office, London.

Doyal, L. (1995) *What Makes Women Sick. Gender and the political economy of health.* Macmillan Press, Basingstoke.

Dutton, D. B. (1988) *Worse Than the Disease. Pitfalls of Medical Progress.* Cambridge University Press, Cambridge.

Fenwick, T. & Parsons, J. (1998) Boldly solving the world: a critical analysis of problem-solving learning as a method of professional education. *Studies in the Education of Adults.* **30,** 53–66.

Fletcher, J. (2000) Some implications for nurses and managers of recent changes to the processing and hearing of medical negligence claims. *Journal of Nursing Management.* **8,** 133–140.

Foucault, M. (1991) *The Birth of the Clinic.* Routledge, London.

Gamarnikow, E. (1978) Sexual division of labor: the case of nursing. In:

*Classic Texts in Health Care* (eds L. Mackay, K. Soothill & K, Melia) (1998), pp. 185–190. Butterworth Heinemann, Oxford.

Goodyear, R. (2000) The nurse practitioner in the US. In: *Nursing Practice, Policy and Change* (ed. M. Gott), pp. 93–113. Radcliffe Medical Press, Oxford.

Gott, M. (ed.) (2000) *Nursing Practice, Policy and Change.* Radcliffe Medical Press, Oxford.

Gøtzche, P. C. & Olsen, O. (2000) Is screening for breast cancer with mammography justifiable? *The Lancet.* **355**, 129–133.

Hartley, J. B. & Woodward, D. (eds) (1987) *The History of Cartography*, Vol 1. University of Chicago Press, Chicago.

Illich, I. (1990) *Limits to Medicine. Medical nemesis: the expropriation of health.* Penguin, London.

Leape, L. L., Brennan, T. A., Laird, N. M., Lawthers, A. G., Localio, A. R., Barnes, B. A., Herbert, L., Newhouse, J. P., Weiler, P. C. & Hiatt, H. (1991) The nature of adverse events in hospitalized patients. Results of the Harvard Medical Practice study II. *New England Journal of Medicine.* **324**, 377–384.

Leape, L. (1999) Error in medicine. In: *Medical Mishaps: Pieces of the Puzzle* (eds M. M. Rosenthal, L. Mulcahy & S. Lloyd-Bostock), pp. 20–38. Open University Press, Buckingham.

Mackay, L. (1993) *Conflicts in Care. Medicine and nursing.* Chapman & Hall, London.

Mackay, L., Soothill, K. & Melia, K. (eds) (1998) *Classic Texts in Health Care.* Butterworth Heinemann, Oxford.

Ritchie Report (2000) *Report of the Inquiry into Quality and Practice Within the National Health Service Arising from the Actions of Rodney Ledward.* Department of Health, London.

Sharpe, V. A. & Faden, A. I. (1998) *Medical Harm: Historical, conceptual and ethical dimensions of iatrogenic illness.* Cambridge University Press, Cambridge.

Styrud, J., Erikson, S., Segelman, J. & Granstrom, L. (1999) Diagnostic accuracy in 2,351 patients undergoing appendicectomy for suspected acute appendicitis: a retrospective study 1986–1993. *Digestive Surgery.* **16**, 39–44

Sweet, S. J. & Norman, I. J. (1995) The doctor–nurse relationship: a selective literature review. *Journal of Advanced Nursing.* **22**, 165–170.

Taylor, S. & Field, D. (eds) (1997) *Sociology of Health and Health Care*, 2nd edn. Blackwell Science, Oxford.

Turnbull, D. (1993) *Maps are Territories, Science is an Atlas.* University of Chicago Press, Chicago.

Twigg, J. & Aitkin, K. (1994) *Carers Perceived: Policy and practice in informal care.* Open University Press, Buckingham.

Vincent, C., Neale, G. & Woloshynowych, M. (2001) Adverse events in British hospitals: preliminary retrospective record review. *British Medical Journal.* **322**, 517–519.

Walsh, M. (2000) *Nursing Frontiers, Accountability and the Boundaries of Care.* Butterworth Heinemann, Oxford.

Whittle, B. & Ritchie, J. (2000) *Prescription for Murder. The true story of mass murderer Dr Harold Frederick Shipman.* Warner Books, London.

Wicks, D. (1998) *Nurses and Doctors at Work: Re-thinking professional boundaries.* Open University Press, Buckingham.

Williams, A. (2000) *Nursing, Medicine and Primary Care.* Open University Press, Buckingham.

Wilson, R., Runciman, W. B., Gibberd, R. W., Harrison, B. T., Newby, L. & Hamilton, J. D. (1995) The quality in Australian health care study. *Medical Journal of Australia.* November, **163**, 458–471.

Woods, D. (2000) Estimate of 98,000 deaths from medical errors is too low, says specialist. *British Medical Journal.* **320**, 1362.

# 2. Defining Medicine and the Nature of Iatrogenic Harm

*Frank Milligan*

## Introduction

There is a good deal of historical and contemporary evidence on medical harm, both occurring directly through medical intervention and as a consequence of the systems derived from western medical efforts and influence. This chapter opens by exploring the nature of western medicine, the focus on the physical body and its aims as expressed through particular forms of language/discourse. The chapter then moves on to the concept of iatrogenic harm and the clinical, social and cultural manifestations of this. Clear examples of such harm are given. It is argued that it is not only doctors that 'do harm' and that those working in the health services, both in the state and independent sectors, can be involved. The focus on western medicine here reflects its influence over much of health care.

## Western medicine – the world-view of a profession

The task of arguing for a clear view of medical harm involves the need to face up to the difficulties of being lucid about the nature of western medicine. The ascendancy of western medicine can be traced back to the seventeenth and eighteenth centuries in terms of the increasing emphasis given to the biological body (Foucault, 1991). This view began to dominate at the expense of other explanations of health and disease. Although a wide range of views on the latter still exist today, an essential difference is that they are labelled by western medicine as alternative and/or complementary. This is an expression of the power of medicine as a profession (Saks, 1998). The efforts of medicine throughout the nineteenth century allowed it to organise itself into a discrete occupation that could claim to be a profession. This required, amongst other things, limited entry and a limited number of practitioners, a specification of minimal educational requirements, and the construction of a code of conduct. Through such mechanisms a distinction could be drawn between doctors, that distinct social group with professional status and others, for example so called quacks (Sharpe & Faden, 1998).

Using historical evidence from the USA, Sharpe and Faden point out that the consolidation of medicine as a profession shifted loyalty away from the patient towards the profession and its key social institution, the hospital. Freidson has argued that the special status of profession, which is ostensibly created to serve the public, carries with it disadvantages:

> 'Once the profession forms such a self-sustaining perspective, protected from others' perspectives, insulated from the necessity of justifying itself to outsiders, it cannot reasonably be expected to see itself and its mission with clear eyes, nor can it reasonably be expected to assume the perspective of its clientele.'
>
> Freidson, 1988 p. 173

The status of profession may therefore lead to a lack of self critique (by the profession). However, one of the advantages the shift in loyalty can bring is security and support to the members of the profession who are frequently involved in precarious and difficult work – the demands of modern health care.

There is no doubt that western medicine dominates the formal aspects of modern health care. There are, of course, parts of the world where this is not true: there are other types of medicine, but the contribution of other health practices is frequently measured against western medicine (Saks, 1994). The term 'western medicine' is used in this book to differentiate it from other forms of medicine and to emphasise its historical roots which lie in so-called western society. Many of those other health practices are given the labels of alternative or complementary, which establishes a distance between that which is scientific and that which, from the medical perspective, is seen as not (Zola, 1975; Saks, 1998). Such a distinction, as will be shown, has some meaning but is also too simplistic. Western medicine is not a single project or a coherent discourse, but has operated in a way that perpetuates a world-view that dominates much of the thinking on health care. It is pervasive and infiltrates our lives in an almost invisible manner (Zola, 1975). It is also inextricably linked to key elements of society, such as government and aspects of industry, such as drug companies (Dutton, 1988).

## The body and the 'gaze'

An integral part of the medical profession to which new members must be initiated is the biomedical perspective. In contrasting medicine with complementary therapies Saks (1998) notes that medicine is based upon an approach that seeks to repair (or remove) those parts that are malfunctioning. Although more recently, claims have been made with regard to a more holistic stance being taken in western medicine (see for example Balint, 1996), Saks claims that notions of mind and spirit remain peripheral to most of its practice. Stewart *et al.* (1995) writing from within medicine, and using experience from a decade of research and education in Canada, argue that the conventional biomedical approach actually ignores the person.

This discrete view of the person as a biological body requires further explanation. An important contribution in this area has been made by Michel Foucault. It is difficult to categorise Foucault and his work, especially as he shunned such classification (Sheridan, 1990), but his writings remain highly influential and are heavily cited in a variety of fields including most of the social sciences, and indeed medicine (Armstrong, 1983). The concept *gaze* figures strongly in one of Foucault's most famous works, *The Birth of the Clinic* (1991) which explored the changes in medicine at the turn of the eighteenth century, changes that laid the foundations of western medicine. It opens with the lines: 'This book is about space, about language, and about death; it is about the act of seeing, the gaze' (Foucault, 1991 p. ix). Gaze as a concept, within this context, is used to explain the historical importance of post-mortem dissection and anatomical anatomy, and how this came to dominate the western medical view of the body:

'For us the human body defines by natural right, the space of origin and of distribution of disease: a space whose lines, volumes, surfaces, and routes are laid down, in accordance with a now familiar geometry, by the anatomical atlas. But this order of the solid, visible body is only one way – in all likelihood neither the first, nor the most fundamental – in which one spatializes disease. There have been, and will be, other distributions of illness.'

Foucault, 1991 p. 3

This points to the fact that other explanations of disease have existed and of course still do exist in other systems, for example Chinese medicine and lay beliefs on health (Taylor & Field, 1997). Perhaps more importantly it also suggests that the western medical view will no doubt continue to change in the future.

Medicine, in the eighteenth century, was seen to have forged a particular view of the human body and its relationship with disease:

> 'What was fundamentally invisible is suddenly offered to the brightness of the gaze, in a movement of appearance so simple, so immediate that it seems to be the natural consequence of a more highly developed experience. It is as if for the first time for thousands of years, doctors, free at last of theories and chimeras, agreed to approach the object of their experience with the purity of an unprejudiced gaze.'
>
> Foucault, 1991 p. 195

Prior to the eighteenth century, links between the body and disease remained unclear. We now take this linkage of disease to the body and physiological change for granted in western societies. For Foucault, however, this was a profound shift that moved disease from something that inserted itself into the vulnerable person, into a notion of the body itself as ill (McNay, 1994). This is a powerful point and one that explains much of the emphasis in current health care – through observing the body you understand the disease.

Although the focus of the medical gaze is the body, it is a dis-embodied gaze, a clinical gaze (Bloor & McIntosh, 1990) which rarely sees the body as a person. It has been argued that within such a perspective it is simply seen as a collection of organs (Deleuze & Guattari 1984, cited in Fox, 1998). Leder (1992) claims that the shift described by Foucault represented a syntactical reorganisation of disease; a reorganisation of language, a shift that reduced it to a specific form of body: it is not a spiritual body, not a lived body, but a body that is treated as dead even in life. Leder gives the interesting analogy of the patient lying on the examination table, almost naked, silent and still – death like. On a simpler level this helps to explain the rather cold approach to people (so-called patients/clients) often seen in health care settings, an approach that is frequently imper-sonal because of this biomedical focus.

The actions of doctors at the Bristol Royal Infirmary are perhaps a recent example of this view being seen in the behaviour of medical staff (Bristol Royal Infirmary Inquiry, 2001). Following controversy over high mortality rates in children undergoing complex heart surgery this English hospital was then subject to a second scandal involving the removal of organs from babies post mortem, often without any consent from the parents (Kennedy, 2000). In viewing the children as a body of organs, it was arguably logical for medical staff to remove some of those organs for research purposes. However, it is evident from the report that the parents viewed their children differently, more as a lived body (person) that should be treated as such, even after death. Parents who had consented were unaware that tissue removal frequently meant complete organ removal, and organs such as the heart carry a symbolic status beyond that of composition, weight, and clinical pathology.

Another practical and powerful example of the gaze is reflected in the emphasis given to the wide range of scans and tests which seek to view and quantify the body and its perceived problems. Spitzack (1992) uses the terms 'gazing apparatuses' to describe the increasing number of these which, since the rise of post-mortem dissection, have been used to create an increasingly 'transparent' body. This is important as so much of medicine and health care is about visualising and quantifying the physical body, yet seeing anatomy through the plethora of tests and scans now available does not necessarily lead to positive health outcomes.

## Limitations of this gaze

A study by Rhodes *et al.* (1999) which interviewed people with chronic low back pain is a good example of the reliance upon visible bodily changes. Those in the study with back pain found that without a discrete anomaly, as might be found in one or more of the many tests they commonly went through, the doctors would not take their back pain seriously. They were themselves reassured when a test actually showed a problem, even though it might be quite serious, as the doctor was then more likely to believe them. The fact that it could be seen, was visible to the gaze, made their pain medically legitimate. However, Rhodes *et al.* concluded that the diagnostic imaging tests often failed to provide a meaningful diagnosis or solution for the person suffering chronic back pain.

A study by Jensen *et al.* (1994) showed that anatomical anomalies of the lower spine are actually quite common in people without back pain. Magnetic resonance imaging (MRI) was undertaken on 98 people who were asymptomatic – had no back pain and had no significant history of back pain. The images obtained were studied by two experienced neuroradiologists and scans from people with symptoms were mixed with the sample. The results showed that

52% of the people without back pain had a disc bulge at at least one level of the lumbar spine and 27% had a disc protrusion. It was concluded that the findings of bulges or protrusions in people with back pain might frequently be coincidental. The authors cited other research, including post-mortem examination studies that demonstrated that asymptomatic abnormalities of the spine are relatively common. It appears that such anomalies, some of which are quite severe, are common in people who do not complain of associated symptoms. Rarely is this comparatively common presence of such anatomical anomalies acknowledged in health care.

As Zajicek (1995) points out, one of the key dilemmas medicine faces is that it may be able to specify 'how' to treat, but it generally fails to decide correctly 'when' to treat. Zajicek argues that the mechanistic, reductionist approach dominant in medical research is itself harmful, iatrogenic. These claims are explored in more depth in the following sections. Of course, the distinction between so called normal and abnormal is even more of a problem in the field of mental health/psychiatry.

Although the medical gaze appears to be genuine, even obvious as we can all see internal anatomy during surgery, for Foucault the gaze is anything but unprejudiced. It is directly linked to the generation of a particular range of language/discourse, and therefore knowledge. Foucault points out that a distinct approach to the body and its health problems is generated through medical language. In fact, little is certain in relation to the body. Even introductory texts on the body as a sociological concept, such as that by Cavallaro (1998), show that there is a complex range of theories relevant to making sense of our bodies. Our bodies, the way we look and feel about them, the manner in which we describe for example what is disabled, are all constructed through our social experience of bodies and what is perceived as being relevant to them.

Lawler (1991) offers a useful example of how such notions can be applied to nursing practice. Her research showed that within general nursing we tend to ignore and as she put it, 'hide behind the screens', a whole range of issues in relation to dealing with other people's bodies. Therefore, although the body is seen as a complex area of study in sociology and philosophy, the approach of both medicine and nursing is discrete, comparatively simplistic and closely focused. The body, and biomedical notions of disease are represented and perpetuated through a particular use of language and words within that language. To take this argument further it is now necessary to explore the concept of discourse.

## Discourse – talking medicine

Discourse refers to language, the content of language and the way in which language is used. Burr (1995) refers to it as a particular picture that is painted of an event or persons through language. Different discourses will describe the same event in different ways; they will have distinct ways of representing the world. Every occupation has what is commonly called its own language. Within professions this is a more contained process in which the student is introduced through training and education to this language, the new words that they must learn, the relationships between these and usage. Student nurses are familiar with this through their early struggles in report/hand-over in which one set of nursing staff give relevant information to the new staff coming on duty, they often find they do not understand many of the terms being used. Discourse however, is not just about words, it is also about the significance given to those words and the ideas that they represent. Through language we, literally, construct our world-view.

It is common in hospital wards to hear a list of medical conditions, both past and present, expressed in relation to a particular person or patient in the nursing report/hand-over. However, these may have little to do with the actual care the person receives (sometimes they will of course be central to the care and support the person requires). So why is such language used even when it might do little to structure the care a person requires? The answer is that nurses, like others in health care, use the discourse with which they are familiar and which appears to make sense within the context within which it is being used. This discourse (the language used) is medically dominated, and so we talk of the patient with atrial fibrillation, chronic lymphatic leukaemia, schizophrenia etc. even though the individual's ability to walk, cook, and communicate their needs effectively might be the priorities. The consequences of these conditions in the acute phases of illness may have a profound impact on the person's health, but once managed they may have little relevance but remain labels used to describe their needs.

Western medicine has generated a discourse that maintains a specific view of people and emphasises certain interventions over others. People are reduced to patients or clients and talked about in particular ways. Naidoo and Wills (1995), writing in relation to health promotion, argue that the discourse of medicine can be described as *biomedical, mechanistic, reductionist* and *allopathic*. By this they mean that people are viewed and treated rather like biological machines. Making sense of this machine involves a process in which ever smaller aspects of the body are examined in isolation – reductionism. The term allopathic refers to a reliance on a system of opposites. An example of this was given above; there is the normal anatomy of the spine and then abnormalities that supposedly cause disease. However, as the evidence from Jensen *et al.* (1994) on lumbar spine anomalies shows, such a simplistic distinction does not always work. The concept of health cannot accurately be separated out into the simplistic categories of the normal and the pathological (Zajicek, 1995).

## The dominant discourse of western medicine

As Turner (1995) points out, in a sociological examination of medical power and knowledge, health care discourse is indeed dominated by medicine. The framework described above by Naidoo and Wills (1995) is helpful but does not adequately embrace the diversity seen in western medicine. Some doctors, as well as some aspects of health care, seem to personify such a world-view, whilst others remain flexible and open to the subtleties of the psychosocial ramifications of various health problems. Further-more, this framework does not seem to encompass some of the more holistic and caring claims made in much of nursing (for example Johns & Freshwater, 1998).

Wicks (1998), using evidence from her research into the shifting nature of doctor–nurse boundaries, offers a more complex view of discourse as found in health care. Her work reflects a range of issues raised here and applies them more specifically within the doctor–nurse relationship. She suggests that although medicine and nur-sing have their own histories, they were almost grafted together through developments in the nineteenth century, including the rise of the teaching hospital. She offers five themes to explain the his-torical development of the current relationship between medicine and nursing.

The first is *discourses of domination*, which arose from the scientific revolution of the seventeenth century. This is reflected in the research methods of western medicine which largely rely upon observable, experimental changes – empirical science. This leads to the second theme in which bodies are seen as *machines*; a mechan-istic perspective that influences diagnosis and research. The third theme is that of *connectedness* or *organicism/holism*. This theme represents the efforts of those that oppose the notion of 'mechanical man'. Wicks (1998) gives evidence to show that such opposition goes back as far as the seventeenth century and arose in resistance

24

to the first two themes she describes. The fourth theme, of *bedside medicine*, describes a situation in which the doctor responds to the patient's expressed wishes. Power in this relationship resides with the patient, a position that was changed through the professionalisation of medicine (Freidson, 1988; Sharpe & Faden, 1998). The last theme is that of *institutional arrangements* that impeded the autonomy of nurses and inhibited their practice of bedside healing.

The work of Wicks is particularly interesting as it brings together several of the arguments made here, especially in relation to the power of discourse in the context of the nurse–doctor relationship. Although the dominant discourse within western medicine is that of scientific, mechanistic reductionism – put simply, approaching people and disease as quantifiable machines and their dysfunctions, there are alternatives. Doctors and others within health care may not always display and perpetuate the gaze described by Foucault or the framework given by Naidoo and Wills, but those efforts are representative of discourses subordinate to the dominant discourse. Their arguments are less important than those within the dominant discourse. It is therefore appropriate to suggest that medicine is not a cohesive project as there is a degree of diversity. This diversity can be seen in day to day health care, and in the practice of some doctors, or perhaps most doctors on some occasions, but the context within which such practices take place is dominated by scientific, mechanistic, reductionism – the dominant discourse of western medicine. This discourse impacts upon the aims of modern health care, because of the historical and contemporary influence of western medicine.

## Iatrogenesis and iatrogenic harm

Having sketched out the aims and influence of western medicine it is now possible to explore the harm that occurs in medically influenced health care. The term iatrogenesis literally means, 'doctor generated' disease and illness (D'Arcy & Griffin, 1986), *iatros* being the Greek word for physician and *genesis*, meaning origin (Illich, 1990). Iatrogenic is defined in the *Oxford English Dictionary* (Second edition 1989) as:

> 'Induced unintentionally by a physician through his diagnosis, manner, or treatment; of or pertaining to the induction of (mental or bodily) disorders, symptoms etc, in this way.'

This is a useful definition although some harm has an intentional aspect to it. Sharpe and Faden (1998) note that the notion of medical harm seems somewhat paradoxical, as our expectation is that medicine will improve rather than diminish our health. Some, such as Rosenthal *et al.* (1999) ignore the terms completely even though their rather politely titled book, *Medical Mishaps*, deals specifically with the realities of medical harm. Similarly, the journalist McTaggart (1996) in her book *What Doctors Don't Tell You*, which covered a wide range of potential problems created through medical treatment, does not once use the terms iatrogenesis or iatrogenic harm.

One of the most interesting and controversial authors to write on iatrogenic harm was Ivan Illich. He used the term iatrogenesis as the name for this new, harmful epidemic of disabling medical control. Although his work was written in the 1970s it is used here as it gives some indication of the potential scale and diversity of iatrogenesis (Illich, 1990). The focus of much of his writing was what he termed, 'The age of Disabling Professions' (Illich *et al.*, 1992 p. 11). Like others writing in the 1970s (for example Zola and McKnight, in Illich *et al.*, 1992) he was concerned with the perceived disabling nature of professions and the institutions with which they are associated. This disabling takes place from behind a mask of service in that the services offered by a profession could reduce the abilities of individuals to cope with particular life events. This also has the effect of making individuals reliant upon professionals, a circle that advantages the profession. The following quotation is representative of the breadth and nature of Illich's critique;

> 'The threat which current medicine represents to the health of populations is analogous to the threat which the volume and intensity of traffic represents to mobility, the threat which education and the media represent to learning, and the threat which urbanization represents to home making.'
>
> Illich, 1990 p. 15

Although Illich has offered a useful framework for clarifying the nature and extent of iatrogenesis, his outspoken style allowed a marginalisation of his work by individuals and professional groups that found it uncomfortable. Horrobin commented in a book titled, *Medical Hubris; A Reply to Ivan Illich*, that '... the silence in the medical world has been deafening' (Horrobin, 1978 p. 2) that little response was made to Illich. One of the interesting things about Horrobin's book is the acceptance of many of Illich's arguments even though it sought to defend medicine. Horrobin conceded that the contribution of medicine to health was overestimated: 'The great changes in the patterns of disease are primarily related to changes in the environment, in the nutritional status of a population, in the supply of clean water and in the effective disposal of excreta' (Horrobin, 1978 p. 9).

Morgan *et al.* (1985) also make it clear that factors such as sanitation, housing and nutrition have a more significant impact on health than medicine. Such arguments are now generally accepted (Taylor & Field, 1997) although sometimes overlooked by both the public and health care workers. It was however openly accepted by the newly elected UK Labour government in 1997 who, in an action plan for tackling poor health, claimed they rejected the old arguments of the past (a reference to the previous Conservative administration) and believed that, '...the **social, economic and environmental** factors tending towards poor health are potent' (DoH, 1999 p. ix (original emphasis)). We wait to see whether this change of stance brings tangible health benefits.

Three forms of harm were described by Illich: *clinical, social,* and *cultural* iatrogenesis.

## Clinical iatrogenesis

Clinical iatrogenesis involves harm through errors, misdiagnosis, and the consequences of some of the prescribed treatments used. Illich specifically identified doctor-inflicted injuries, unnecessary surgery, useless treatments such as antibiotic therapy for viral infections, and claimed;

> 'The pain, dysfunction, disability and anguish resulting from technical medical intervention now rival the morbidity due to traffic and industrial accidents and even war-related activities, and make the impact of medicine one of the most rapidly spreading epidemics of our time.'
>
> Illich, 1990 p. 35

One of the interesting points linked to this claim is the notion of risk. Once reasonable standards of sanitation, nutrition and housing have been achieved, so the risk of ill health from other factors increases, and this invariably includes western medicine and the health systems it dominates.

## Social iatrogenesis

Illich claimed that western medicine not only harms through direct aggression against the individual as described above, but also through its socio-political power as a profession leading to the medicalisation of much of everyday life. He was particularly concerned with the monopoly medicine seeks to hold over health. This is evident in the power and control it is able to wield in relation to access to the sick role (gate-keeping) and repression of other forms of health-seeking activity. Within the sphere of social iatrogenesis Illich focused on the institutionalisation of health care; '... when all suffering is "hospitalized" and homes become inhospitable to birth, sickness, and death...', and continued, '... or when suffering, mourning, and healing outside the patient role are labelled a form of deviance' (Illich, 1990 p. 49). He claimed that mutual care and self-medication are turned into crimes. For Illich, death itself was an enemy of medicine, one that it seeks to defeat. He used the term 'death under intensive care' and was particularly scathing of medicine on this matter:

> 'Like all other major rituals of industrial society, medicine in practice takes the form of a game. The chief function of the physician becomes that of an umpire. He is the agent or representative of the social body, with the duty to make sure that everyone plays the game according to the rules. The rules, of course, forbid leaving the game and dying in any fashion that has not been specified by the umpire. Death no longer occurs except as the self-fulfilling prophecy of the medicine man.'
>
> Illich, 1990 p. 208

Illich, like others, maintained that medicine has gained a quasi-religious status (Zola, 1975). He also explored the moral enterprise within medicine: that it frequently defines what is normal, proper and desirable and creates a new group of outsiders with each new diagnosis. He asserted that medicine categorises, amongst others, those who can drive a car; stay away from work; be locked up; become soldiers; cross borders; become prostitutes and commit crime. Medicine defines who is dead and what type of death they had (Illich, 1990). This power to categorise has also been commented on by Foucault (1991) and is explored here in several of the later chapters.

## Cultural iatrogenesis

The third form of medical harm described was cultural iatrogenesis. 'It sets in when the medical enterprise saps the will of people to suffer their reality' (Illich, 1990 p. 133). Medicine was seen to overturn the cultural experiences that define self-care and suffering;

'Wherever in the world a culture is medicalized, the traditional framework of habits that can become conscious in the personal practices of the virtue of hygiene is progressively trammelled by a mechanical system, a medical code by which individuals submit to the instructions emanating from hygienic custodians.'

Illich, 1990 p. 137

In other words, individuals are distanced from their own culture and disabled by reliance upon the imposed, mechanistic pseudo-culture of medicine. Those living in western societies are born into a culture which represents medical influence. The notion of cultural iatrogenesis helps to explain the resistance of western medicine to alternative and complementary therapies in that it is attempting to devalue potential competitors. The rise of these, despite this resistance (Saks, 1994; 1998), is perhaps a reflection of the need to find coping mechanisms for illness and disease, frequently from quite different cultures, e.g. Chinese medicine, to replace those which have been 'trammelled' by medicine. This diversity might also be an example of globalisation and the increasing cultural diversity that seems to go with this (Giddens, 1990). It is also clear that Illich felt that a degree of suffering, of pain and discomfort, was part of being human.

## Recent evidence on iatrogenic harm

### Clinical iatrogenesis

Clear evidence in relation to Illich's claims of clinical iatrogenesis can be found more recently. For example, in the USA it has been estimated that between 44,000 and 98,000 deaths a year are caused by medical error (Kohn *et al.*, 2000). The calculations made in the report to the US federal government were used to claim that medical errors were the eighth commonest cause of death, listed above road traffic accidents, breast cancer and HIV/AIDS. One of the editors of the report subsequently alleged that even the top end figure of 98,000 was an underestimate as it only included inpatients and not those being treated out in the community (Woods, 2000). The Harvard Medical Practice studies (Brennan *et al.*, 1991; Leape, 1991), which have been the basis for other research into adverse events and negligence in the UK (Vincent *et al.*, 2001) and Australia (Wilson *et al.*, 1995), concluded that there was a substantial amount of injury caused to patients from medical management. These studies were used to help estimate the total possible number of deaths on NHS hospitals from preventable adverse events, a figure that could be as high as 25,000 a year (Bristol Royal Infirmary Inquiry, 2001). Again, deaths from adverse events that occur in the community, as opposed to within NHS premises, are unlikely to be included in this figure. It therefore underestimates the total number of deaths from this cause in the UK. The relevance of these studies should not be underestimated, particularly as they are acknowledged as accurate and substantial pieces within the medical community and were accepted by the Bristol Inquiry team.

The National Audit Commission estimates that around 5,000 people a year are dying of hospital acquired infections in England (Comptroller & Auditor General, 2000). Another example includes unnecessary and inappropriate surgery, both of which have been analysed in some depth by Sharpe and Faden (1998). They take the view that surgery is in itself a harm but is, when used appropriately, a necessary harm that should improve, or lead to more accurate diagnosis of, the patient's condition. In consenting to surgery, '...the patient accepts actual and potential harm only in anticipation of some greater identified clinical benefit to be gained' (Sharpe & Faden, 1998 p. 208). A distinction is drawn between unnecessary surgery and the more recent usage of the concept appropriateness: 'The appropriateness of a surgical procedure is not *simply* a function of its expectation of net clinical benefit to the patient but also of the way in which benefit is understood and valued by patients and others in the decision-making process' (Sharpe and Faden, 1998 p. 202 (original emphasis)). A number of studies from the US are summarised and some are reproduced here in Table 2.1. These figures show the levels of unnecessary or inappropriate surgery found within explicit criteria studies estimating unnecessary and inappropriate surgery.

It can be seen that a significant amount of surgery is questionable in terms of need. A variety of factors are used to explain why people may be subject to surgery that is clinically useless or non-beneficial, but it is concluded that the key problems lie in the generation, dissemination and application of medical knowledge. In addition to these examples the number of normal appendixes removed when inflammatory disease is suspected has been found to be anywhere between 25% (Styrud *et al.*, 1999) and 41% (Mosley, 1999).

The case of Rodney Ledward, a UK gynaecologist who was removed from the medical register in 1998, gives another perspective on the concepts of unnecessary and inappropriate surgery (Ritchie Report, 2000). The report chronologically describes the vagaries of his practice from 1980 to 1996 using a variety of witnesses including the patients themselves, various levels of medical

**Table 2.1** Explicit criteria studies addressing unnecessary or inappropriate procedures. (Sharpe & Faden, 1998 p. 204. Reproduced in part, with permission from Cambridge University Press. The references for these studies* are cited in the original text)

| Year | Procedure | Unnecessary/ inappropriate | Number |
|------|-----------|----------------------------|--------|
| 1977* | Tonsillectomy | 86% | 3072 |
| 1987* | Gastrointestinal endoscopy | 17% | 1585 |
| 1988* | Carotid endarterectomy | 32% | 1302 |
| 1991* | Carotid endarterectomy | 17% | 2200 |
| 1988* | Pacemaker | 20% | 382 |
| 1988* | Coronary artery bypass graft | 14% | 386 |
| 1993* | Coronary artery bypass graft | 2% | 1388 |
| 1993* | Coronary angiography | 4% | 1355 |
| 1990* | Hysterectomy | 8% | 257 |
| 1993* | Hysterectomy | 16% | 642 |

staff, through to nurses, some of his secretaries and a number of senior managers. In addition to the significant numbers of surgical errors he made throughout this timespan, it is clear that he also performed a substantial amount of unnecessary surgery. Comments such as '... *we express our concern as to whether all these procedures were medically necessary*' (Ritchie Report, 2000 p. 90, original emphasis) occur repeatedly in the report.

Ledward actively encouraged many women to be seen privately instead of as NHS patients. The evidence in the report suggests that this was a dangerous shift for them as unnecessary surgery was more common amongst his private patients. Surgery for financial gain is an old problem in medicine, especially in the USA with its fee-for-service systems (Sharpe & Faden, 1998). Some might seek to devalue the relevance of the evidence in the Ledward report on the grounds that he was a maverick, an isolated case. However, his levels of surgery and propensity to undertake total hysterectomies even on young women, were not dissimilar enough to those of his colleagues for staff to raise significant concerns earlier in his career. Furthermore, his status as a consultant dissuaded other staff from raising their concerns (see Chapters 3 and 4 for further discussion on the potential influence of status on harm generation).

## Social iatrogenesis

In terms of social iatrogenesis, the book *Cyborg Babies* (Davis-Floyd & Dumit, 1998) is a more recent example of sociological criticism with regard to the invasion of life, in this case from pre-conception, through childbirth to neonates, by medicine. It shows how much of what might once have loosely been called natural, has become technical, controlled and subject to the surveillance of health care professionals and their machines. Indeed, Mentor (1998) goes further and argues that home birth has been criminalised by medicine in western society.

Another example of social iatrogenesis is the expansion of mass screening programmes, interventions that inevitably impact upon the everyday lives of the public. The article by Quinn *et al.* (1999a) is an example of the complexity of the arguments in terms of substantiating such programmes. Their study compared age-specific mortality on cervical cancer before and after the introduction of the national call and recall system in Great Britain. They concluded that without screening there might have been a further 800 deaths from cervical cancer in women under 55. However, they acknowledged that the programme does not meet the two most important criteria for screening programmes laid down by the World Health Organisation: the disease is relatively uncommon and its natural course is not well understood. Commenting on the findings of the Quinn *et al.* study, Vaidya and Baum (1999) calculated, using the original data, that mortality could be shown to have increased for some age groups of women during the time scale quoted. Quinn *et al.* (1999b) responded by stating that there was conclusive evidence that cervical screening had reduced both incidence and mortality. However, they also reiterated their concerns with regard to the test having low sensitivity and specificity, and the fact that many tests are technically unsatisfactory, something subsequently supported by the audit described below (Ferriman, 2001). Adab *et al.* (1999) argue that the work of Quinn *et al.* shows that a reduction in mortality from cervical cancer in Hong Kong could be achieved if a centralised screening programme were to be initiated there. Interestingly, they also note that harm is being caused through the unnecessary screening of women at low risk.

A recent example of the continuing problems associated with cervical screening comes from the findings of an audit into test accuracy in Leicestershire. This found that of the 403 women who had developed cervical cancer between the years of 1993 and 2000, only 79 had not been for regular smear tests. In 122 of the remaining 324 cases an error had been made by the screeners who reported the slide results. Of these 122 women, 78 experienced a worsening of their condition before it was diagnosed and 14 died (Ferriman, 2001). It was noted that this audit was probably representative of the situation in other cervical screening centres throughout the UK (Boseley, 2001). Leicestershire was not chosen because it had a known problem, but because an experienced team of clinicians wanted to review and thereby improve their standards (Ferriman, 2001).

Similar controversy can be found in relation to both mammography and bone density screening. With regard to the former, Wright and Mueller (1995) examined the results of six studies on the effectiveness of mammography. They noted that early studies that had claimed significant benefits from breast screening had led to strong professional and public support for such programmes. However, there had been little publicity about subsequent trials showing little or no benefit in any age group. They concluded:

> 'Since the benefit achieved is marginal, the harm caused is substantial, and the costs incurred are enormous, we suggest that public funding for breast cancer screening in any age group is not justifiable.'
>
> Wright & Mueller, 1995 p. 29

They agreed with others at the time, that the cost of each life saved through screening mammography was £558,000 (US$1.2 million).

More recently, Gøtzsche and Olsen (2000) reported on a study that revisited previous Swedish trials on breast screening and a meta-analysis of relevant research including studies from other countries. Like Wright and Mueller (1995) they concluded 'Screening for breast cancer with mammography is unjustified' (Gøtzsche & Olsen, 2000 p. 129). This caused a storm of debate in the UK, within both the media and medicine. One of the most important aspects of this controversy involved the Cochrane Breast Cancer Group (CBCG) which reviewed the evidence from the Gøtzsche and Olsen study in preparation for publication within the Cochrane Collaboration. Such publication infers that the systematic review is of a higher quality than a review completed according to non-Cochrane protocols (Horton, 20001). However, the CBCG changed significant aspect of the report compiled by Gøtzsche and Olsen (Olsen & Gøtzsche, 2001), a report based upon their original data and subsequent revision of that work in response to criticisms made of it. This led Horton (2001) to claim, in a commentary on these events in *The Lancet*, that the CBCG had interfered with academic freedom.

In that same edition of the journal Olsen and Gøtzsche (2001) comment on the Cochrane review response to their submission by including, amongst other points, evidence that screening leads to more aggressive treatment, and this includes treatments for histological cancer that is biologically benign. In other words, some women are being treated for cancer, as they have this particular type of breast malignancy, although it will probably do them little harm within their lifetime. Mammography is likely to detect such lesions. The official position in the UK remains one supportive of breast screening by mammography (DoH, 2001), a stance supported by experts at the World Health Organisation who were brought together in an attempt to end uncertainty on this matter. The 24 experts from 11 countries concluded that mammography does reduce the chance of dying from breast cancer in women aged 50–69 (Kmietowicz, 2002).

Bone density screening is not as widespread as the programmes described above, but again evidence in relation to its effectiveness is mixed. Sheldon *et al.* (1996) suggest that screening bone density (usually in post-menopausal women) is unreliable and expensive but note that pressures exist to introduce such measures. A meta-analysis of studies from 1985 to 1994 by Marshall *et al.* (1996) concluded that measurement of bone mineral density could predict fracture risk but could not identify individuals who will have a fracture. Commenting on an advisory group report made to the Department of Health supporting the use of such screening, Sheldon *et al.* (1996, p. 297) ask '... whose interest will best be served by recommending the increased purchase of bone densitometry and this back door advocacy of screening – the general public or the equipment and pharmaceutical suppliers?'

One final point worth considering in relation to mass screening programmes is that they are usually aimed at women. Doyal (1995), in a book that critically explores the impact of the biomedical model on women's health, argues that although doctors may play an important part in many women's lives, modern medicine is rarely the major determinant of their health – other, socio-economic factors are more significant. Although the contribution of these screening programmes to women's health remains contentious, what is clear is the fact that it subjects them to surveillance and portrays aspects of their sexuality as being problematic.

## Cultural iatrogenesis

Finding specific examples of cultural iatrogenesis is difficult, in part because of its pervasive nature – it becomes part of everyday life. By definition it is part of the map of everyday social interaction and relationships. Critique can therefore prove elusive. However, the case of Harold Shipman, the general practitioner (GP) convicted of multiple murder, gives a good insight into this aspect of iatrogenesis. He was initially convicted of 15 murders, but an audit into his practice between 1974 and 1998 which included comparisons with GPs with similar workloads and an analysis of death certificates, concluded that there were 236 excess deaths about which there should be concern (Baker, 2001). Furthermore, excess numbers of deaths were evident from the early years of his practice. The public inquiry into Shipman's practice concluded that he had killed a total of 215 patients. In a further 45 cases there was real cause to suspect that Shipman might have killed the patient with insufficient evidence being available to reach a conclusion in 38 other cases (Smith, 2002).

Comment from those in the local community where Shipman practised showed that many people had their suspicions about his activities but felt unable to report these (Whittle & Ritchie, 2000). For example, a local taxi driver was concerned because his regular fares, the old ladies he took shopping and to the post office to collect their pension, were dying in large numbers if they were Harold Shipman's patients. The routine nature of these trips meant that he and his wife, who kept a list of clients, knew the women well and the link with Shipman became clear. Similarly, the local undertaker noticed that many of Shipman's patients died with their clothes on in easy chairs. This is unusual as elderly people who suffer a medical crisis such as a heart attack or stroke, and die at home, will usually end up on the floor. As with the taxi driver and his wife, the staff in the undertakers felt unable to say anything about their concerns. They doubted their own judgement on the matter, and they doubted that anyone would listen to them if they queried the activities of a doctor, especially one who was well known locally.

This is an example of cultural iatrogenesis in that such extreme harm was able to continue as these people, and other local GPs who had similar suspicions, were disabled by the trust they had in medicine and medical systems. That trust was misplaced in that the profession of medicine failed to identify a renegade practitioner and systems were not in place within the NHS to monitor the death rates and prescription habits of GPs. Shipman killed his victims with an overdose of opiates.

Although the work of Illich, through his three forms of iatrogenic harm, is useful in terms of identifying and quantifying the possible extent of medically influenced harm, it too has its limits. Illich did not offer any clear way forward or alternatives to the problems he so vociferously described.

## *Conclusion*

It has been argued in this chapter that to be clear with regard to the extent of unnecessary harm within modern health provision it is necessary to clarify the nature of western medicine and its influence over health care. Although western medicine comprises a variety of practitioners involved in a range of diverse activities, there are enough similarities in its approach to the definition of disease and its goals in relation to health care to claim that it operates as a dominant discourse. It has been, and continues to be, highly influential in determining the approach taken to a range of health problems and the various systems and policies set in place to deal with these. As a profession, a discrete and self-regulating occupational group, medicine brings with it both advantages and disadvantages. The status of profession helps give doctors the protection and support they need to undertake some of the difficult work inevitably involved in health care, but it also raises the question of whose needs are really being met – those of the patient, or those of the profession and its individual members? Cases like those of Ledward (Ritchie Report, 2000), Shipman (Baker, 2001) and the Bristol Royal Infirmary Inquiry (2001; DoH, 2002) show it is frequently still the latter.

It has been noted that the most significant improvements to health have historically been achieved through environmental and social changes and this is unlikely to change. This fact is sometimes overlooked in health care systems dominated by western medicine with its emphasis on acute interventions and the biological body. Acute interventions are only a small part of the total work of health care although they are the elements that attract public and media attention. This is convenient for medicine as it perpetuates a social status that it is reluctant to see challenged, but the gaze of medicine is limited and literally body focused. Evidence cited here gives a brief insight into the limits of this perspective and the language, the power of discourse, which maintains this high social status. This poses a particular problem for nursing, as deference to medical opinion may not always lead to the best health outcome. Similarly, in taking over increasing amounts of work previously undertaken by medical staff, nurses may be left exposed as they do not have the same levels of protection as are afforded to the profession of medicine. This point is returned to in the following two chapters.

Iatrogenic harm in its clinical, social and cultural guises, is a diverse and significant health problem and like other threats to health it is necessary for those that claim the enhancement of health as their goal to scrutinise it. It is not just about the harm of errors and unnecessary treatments, it concerns labelling and categorisation and the structuring of social expectations in health care provision. A controversial, but useful example, is breast screening by mammography. The evidence of the effectiveness of this approach, when balanced against the stress, cost and risks to women subject to screening, which includes the unnecessary treatment some will endure (Olsen & Gøtzsche, 2001), is flimsy but a national programme remains in place in the UK. Although substantiating such a programme is reliant upon interpretation of the research evidence, other factors should not be forgotten. Breast screening focuses on the biological body; it subjects women to mass surveillance, utilises technology and perhaps reassures the public in the sense that something is being done. Finally, it is suggested that the term iatrogenesis is appropriate, even though it is acknowledged that all those working in health care may cause and perpetuate unnecessary harm, as too much of health care is literally 'doctor generated'. Iatrogenesis is a framework through which the contribution of medicine and health care can be viewed more clearly and critically. The chapters that follow will help illustrate the limits of some aspects of current health care practice and the negative health effects that can be caused through some practices which are currently considered acceptable.

# References

Adab, P., McGhee, S. & Hedley, A. (1999) Study shows the importance of centralised organisation in screening. *British Medical Journal.* **319**, 642.

Armstrong, D. (1983) *Political Anatomy of the Body; Medical knowledge in Britain in the twentieth century.* Cambridge University Press, Cambridge.

Baker, R. (2001) *Harold Shipman's Clinical Practice 1974–1998.* Department of Health, London.

Balint, J. (1996) Regaining the initiative. Forging a new model of the patient–physician relationship. *Journal of the American Medical Association.* **275**, 887–891.

Bloor, M. & McIntosh, J. (1990) Surveillance and concealment: a comparison of techniques of client resistance in therapeutic communities and health visiting. In: *Readings in Medical Sociology* (eds S. Cunningham-Burley & N. P. McKeganey), pp. 159–181. Tavistock/Routledge, London.

Boseley, S. (2001) Smear tests that failed to save lives. *Guardian.* 4 May, p. 4.

Brennan, T. A., Leape, L. L., Laird, N. M., Hebert, L., Localio, A. R., Lawthers, A. G., Newhouse, J. P., Weiler, P. C. & Hiatt, H. H. (1991) Incidence of adverse events and negligence in hospitalized patients. Results of the Harvard Medical Practice Study I. *New England Journal of Medicine.* **324**, 370–376.

Bristol Royal Infirmary Inquiry (2001) *Learning from Bristol. The report of the public inquiry into children's heart surgery at the Bristol Royal Infirmary, 1984–1995.* Department of Health, London.

Burr, V. (1995) *An Introduction to Social Constructionism.* Routledge, London.

Cavallaro, D. (1998) *The Body for Beginners.* Writers and Readers, New York.

Comptroller and Auditor General (2000) *The Management and Control of Hospital Acquired Infection in Acute NHS Trusts in England.* Department of Health, London.

D'Arcy, P. F. & Griffin, J. P. (1986) *Iatrogenic Diseases*, 3rd edn. Oxford University Press, Oxford.

Davis-Floyd, R. & Dumit, J. (eds) (1998) *Cyborg Babies: From techno sex to techno-tots.* Routledge, New York.

DoH (1999) *Saving Lives: Our healthier nation.* The Stationery Office, London.

DoH (2001) *Cancer – speeding the treatment, slowing the disease.* Available from www.doh.gov.uk

DoH (2002) *Learning from Bristol: The Department of Health's response to the Report of the Public Inquiry into children's heart surgery at the Bristol Royal Infirmary 1984–1995.* The Stationery Office, London

Doyal, L. (1995) *What Makes Women Sick. Gender and the political economy of health.* Macmillan Press, Basingstoke.

Dutton, D. B. (1998) *Worse Than The Disease. Pitfalls of medical progress.* Cambridge University Press, Cambridge.

Ferriman, A. (2001) Audit shows weaknesses in cervical cancer screening. *British Medical Journal.* **322**, 1141.

Foucault, M. (1991) *The Birth of the Clinic.* Routledge, London.

Fox, N. (1998) The promise of postmodernism for the sociology of health and medicine. In: *Modernity, Medicine and Health* (eds G. Scambler & P. Higgs), pp. 29–45. Routledge, London.

Freidson, E. (1988) Profession of medicine: a study of the sociology of applied knowledge. In: *Classic Texts in Health Care* (eds L. Mackay. K. Soothill & K. Melia) (1998), pp. 170–174. Butterworth Heinemann, Oxford.

Giddens, A. (1990) *The Consequences of Modernity.* Stanford University Press, Stanford, CA.

Gøtzsche, P. C. & Olsen, O. (2000) Is screening for breast cancer with mammography justifiable? *The Lancet.* **355**, 129–133.

Horrobin, D. (1978) *Medical Hubris: A reply to Ivan Illich.* Churchill Livingstone, Glasgow.

Horton, R. (2001) Screening mammography – an overview revisited. *The Lancet.* **358**, 1284–1285.

Illich, I. (1990) *Limits to Medicine. Medical nemesis: the expropriation of health.* Penguin, London.

Illich, I., Zola, I. K., McKnight, J., Caplan, J. & Shaiken, H. (1992) *Disabling Professions.* Marion Boyars, New York.

Illich, I. (2001) *Medical Nemesis: The Limits to Medicine.* First published by Marion Boyars Publishers, New York, 1975. Reprinted 2001.

Jensen, M. C., Brant-Zawadzki, M. N., Obuchowski, N., Modic, M. T., Malkasian, D. & Ross, J. S. (1994) Magnetic resonance imaging of the lumbar spine in people without back pain. *New England Journal of Medicine*. **331**, 69–73.

Johns C. & Freshwater D. (eds) (1998) *Transforming Nursing through Reflective Practice*. Blackwell Science, Oxford.

Kennedy, I., Howard, R., Jarman, B. & Maclean, M. (2000) *The Inquiry into the Management of Care of Children Receiving Complex Heart Surgery at The Bristol Royal Infirmary. Interim report – removal and retention of human material*. The Bristol Royal Infirmary, Bristol.

Kmietowicz, Z. (2002) WHO insists screening can cut breast cancer rates. *British Medical Journal*. **324**, 695.

Kohn, L. T., Corrigan, J. M. & Donaldson, M. S. (eds) (2000) *To Err is Human: Building a safer health system*. National Academy Press, Washington DC.

Lawler, J. (1991) *Behind the Screens*. Churchill Livingstone, Melbourne.

Leape, L. L., Brennan, T. A., Laird, N. M., Lawthers, A. G., Localio, A. R., Barnes, B. A., Herbert, L., Newhouse, J. P., Weiler, P. C. & Hiatt, H. (1991) The nature of adverse events in hospitalized patients. Results of the Harvard Medical Practice study II. *New England Journal of Medicine*. **324**, 377–384.

Leder, D. (1992) A tale of two bodies: the Cartesian corpse and the lived body. In: *The Body in Medical Thought and Practice* (ed. D. Leder), pp. 17–35. Kluwer Academic Publishers, Dordrecht.

Marshall, D., Johnell, O. & Wedel, H (1996) Meta-analysis of how measures of bone mineral density predict occurrence of osteoporotic fractures. *British Medical Journal*. **312**, 1254–1259.

McNay, L. (1994) *Foucault: a Critical Introduction*. Continuum, New York.

McTaggart, L. (1996) *What Doctors Don't Tell You: The truth about the dangers of modern medicine*. Thorsons, London.

Mentor, S. (1998) Witches, nurses, midwives, and cyborgs. In: *Cyborg Babies. From Techno Sex to Techno-tots* (eds R. Davis-Floyd & J. Dumit), pp. 67–89. Routledge, New York.

Morgan, M. Calnan, M. & Manning, N. (1985) *Sociological Approaches to Health and Medicine*. Croom Helm, Guildford.

Mosley, J. G. (1999) Has the change in junior doctors' hours resulted in an increased number of appendices being removed? *Annals of the Royal College of Surgeons of England*. **81**, 359–360.

Naidoo, J. & Wills, J. (1995) *Health Promotion: Foundations for practice*. Baillière Tindall, London.

Olsen, O. & Gøtzsche, P. C. (2001) Cochrane review on screening for breast cancer with mammography. *The Lancet*. **358**, 1340–1342

Quinn, M., Babb, P., Jones, J. & Allen, E. (1999a) Effect of screening on incidence of and mortality from cancer of the cervix in England: evaluation based on routinely collected statistics. *British Medical Journal*. **318**, 904–908.

Quinn, M., Babb, P. & Jones, J. (1999b) Authors' reply [to Vaidya & Baum 1999]. *British Medical Journal*. **319**, 642.

Rhodes, L. A., McPhillips-Tangum, C. A., Markham, C. & Klenk, R. (1999) The power of the visible: the meaning of diagnostic tests in chronic back pain. *Social Science and Medicine*. **48**, 1189–1203.

Ritchie Report (2000) *Report of the Inquiry into Quality and Practice Within the National Health Service Arising From the Actions of Rodney Ledward.* Department of Health, London.

Rosenthal, M. M., Mulcahy, L. & Lloyd-Bostock, S. (eds) (1999) *Medical Mishaps: Pieces of the puzzle.* Open University Press, Buckingham.

Saks, M. (1994) The alternatives to medicine. In: *Challenging Medicine* (eds J. Gabe, D. Kelleher & G. Williams), pp. 84–103. Routledge, London.

Saks, M (1998) Medicine and complementary medicine. In: *Modernity, Medicine and Health* (eds G. Scambler & P. Higgs), pp. 198–215. Routledge, London.

Sharpe, V. A. & Faden, A. I. (1998) *Medical Harm: Historical, conceptual, ethical dimensions of iatrogenic illness.* Cambridge University Press, Cambridge.

Sheldon, T. A., Raffle, A. & Watt, I. (1996) Department of Health shoots itself in the hip; why the report on the Advisory Group on Osteoporosis undermines evidence based purchasing. *British Medical Journal*. **312**, 296–298.

Sheridan, A. (1990) *Michel Foucault: The will to truth.* Routledge, London.

Smith, D. J. (2002) *The Shipman Inquiry: Independent public inquiry into the issues arising from the case of Harold Shipman.* Department of Health, London.

Spitzack, C. (1992) Foucault's political body in medical praxis. In: *The Body in Medical Thought and Practice* (ed. D. Leder), pp. 51–68. Kluwer Academic Publishers, Dordrecht.

Stewart, M., Brown, J. B., Weston, W. W., McWhinney, I. R. & McWilliam, C. L. (1995) *Patient-centred medicine: transforming the clinical method.* Sage, Thousand Oaks, California.

Styrud, J., Eriksson, S., Segelman, J. & Granström, L. (1999) Diagnostic accuracy in 2351 patients undergoing appendicectomy for suspected acute appendicitis. A retrospective study 1986–1993. *Digestive Surgery*. **16**, 39–44.

Taylor, S. & Field, D. (eds) (1997) *Sociology of Health and Health Care*, 2nd edn. Blackwell Science, Oxford.

Turner, B. S. (1995) *Medical Power and Social Knowledge*, 2nd edn. Sage, London.

Vaidya, J. S. & Baum, M. (1999) Does screening really reduce mortality? (letter). *British Medical Journal*. **319**, 642.

Vincent, C., Neale, G. & Woloshynowych, M. (2001) Adverse events in British hospitals: preliminary retrospective record review. *British Medical Journal*. **322**, 517–519.

Whittle, B. & Ritchie, J. (2000) *Prescription for Murder. The true story of mass murderer Dr Harold Frederick Shipman.* Warner Books, London.

Wicks, D. (1998) *Nurses and Doctors at Work; Re-thinking professional boundaries.* Open University Press, Buckingham.

Wilson, R., Runciman, W. B., Gibberd, R. W., Harrison, B. T., Newby, L. & Hamilton, J. D. (1995) The quality in Australian health care study. *Medical Journal of Australia.* **163**, 458–471.

Woods, D. (2000) Estimate of 98,000 deaths from medical errors is too low, says specialist. *British Medical Journal.* **320**, 1362.

Wright, C. J. & Mueller, C. B. (1995) Screening mammography and public health policy: the need for perspective. *The Lancet.* **346**, 29–32.

Zajicek, G. (1995) Normative medicine. *Medical Hypotheses.* **45**, 331–334.

Zola, I. (1975) In the name of health and illness: on some socio-political consequences of medical influence. *Social Science and Medicine.* **9**, 83–87.

# 3. Being a Professional – A Defence Against Causing Harm?

*Kate Robinson*

## Introduction

One of the central tenets of this book – and the motivation for its creation – is that as nurses embrace a range of new tasks and as health care becomes more complex, so the potential for nurses to cause harm increases. This is not to say that the work in which nurses have been engaged up until now has not had the potential to cause harm – far from it. An obvious example would be the management of a patient's movement in bed – a function which has always been accepted as central to the role of the nurse. Here, a failure to help a patient who cannot move independently can have catastrophic consequences. However, each new domain of activity which is opened up to nurses, such as drug prescribing, will entail new sets of risks and require new ways of assessing and managing the risk. Furthermore, this expansion of their role comes at a time when there is a greatly increased public awareness of the risks attached to supposedly therapeutic activity and an increasing willingness to hold professionals to account for their actions. Clearly, then, it will be sensible for nurses, both individually and collectively, to consider how they will manage these new risks, and indeed to reflect on how effectively they are managing the risks inherent in their more taken for granted roles.

One of the ways in which other occupations, notably medicine, have attempted to manage the risks involved in their practice is through demanding and securing the status and organisational trappings of a profession. This has the potential to lower risk in a number of ways. The argument in essence is that the profession itself sets standards of competence for initial entry and thereafter guides the conduct of its members through the provision of codes of practice. This is intended to solve the problem for the individual in deciding who might or might not be a safe practitioner and for the state of deciding who is deserving of status and reward and (particularly within a state supported system) of employment. In essence the profession says to the general public: 'you're not competent to know who is a good or bad practitioner because you can't understand the knowledge base, so we'll do the testing and certify the competent ones for you.' Anyone who has tried to employ a good plumber will have some sympathy for the argument, but of course one obvious consequence is that only the profession gets to say what the practitioners should know and do. Nevertheless, this model has been very attractive to nursing and many nurses have been engaged throughout the last century in the drive to professionalise nursing – to emulate the medical profession – and this chapter will explore this aspiration and its potential impact on risk management strategies and the avoidance of mishaps.

The term 'mishaps' has been used in the literature (Rosenthal *et al.*, 1999) to apply to a whole range of events which might individually be labelled as error, negligence, adverse event, mistake, or accident. It is intended to avoid using terms which attribute blame or motivation. Gray (1997) noted that patients were less tolerant of what are euphemistically called 'side effects' than clinicians. One suspects the same may be true of mishaps. Although the desire to protect the public from risk and avoid mishap can be said to be an argument for the promotion of professions, there is the converse, that professional status also has the potential to inhibit the ability to manage risk properly. Moreover, the potential for harm does not depend on whether or not nursing achieves professional status (in practice, it is difficult to see how nursing could attain the type of status which doctors have achieved) but even the aspiration to professionalise may promote strategies for action which pose a risk to the public. The link between professional status and iatrogenesis (see Chapter 2) is complex. In part it relates to the socialisation of individual practitioners into ways of thinking that preclude self awareness; in part it is because peers are required to protect their colleagues from scrutiny or investigation: and in part it is because the profession collectively defines aspects of people's life experience in ways that may be disabling or positively harmful.

## *The professionalisation agenda*

A pervading theme of the history of nursing in the twentieth century is the extent to which the members of the occupation and the employers supported or opposed the proposal that nursing should become a 'proper' profession akin to medicine. Nursing is not unique in this, social work and teaching have experienced similar struggles, and like them nursing is internally divided about the virtues of professionalising (see, for example, Carpenter 1977; White 1985). Abbott and Meerabeau (1988 p. 2) comment: 'Both social work and nursing ... have been concerned to establish their professional status, to develop professionalizing strategies, and both have been divided internally as to whether or not professional status is something desirable and to be striven for.'

Nevertheless, the lobby for professionalisation within nursing was large enough to mount a substantial campaign which was based loosely on the sociological trait theory of professions. A continuing theme in the sociological analysis of professions has been the attempt to define the characteristics of a profession. This depends on the idea that there are certain core traits which particular occupations possess which underpin their claim to be a profession. Definitions of these traits vary between analysts but, in general, they include the ability to:

- control entry to the profession
- define the portfolio of appropriate tasks to be undertaken
- control the boundaries with other occupations
- define the knowledge base.

In addition, professions were assumed to have a service ethic which was manifested through a code of practice or ethics.

The professionalisers' strategy therefore sought to introduce or reinforce these characteristics within nursing in order to underpin the claim for professional status. The creation of the United Kingdom Central Council for Nursing, Midwifery and Health Visiting (UKCC) can be seen as a significant step forward in this, in part because it provided for a single body to regulate the occupation and in part because it provided a focus for these debates to take place. The UKCC, which was replaced by the Nursing and Midwifery Council (NMC) in 2002, has concerned itself with precisely those issues integral to the trait theory – codes of conduct, definition of appropriate tasks, education and role boundaries. (For further discussion of the role of the UKCC and NMC see Chapter 4.)

Another locus of debate was the main union for nurses, the Royal College of Nursing, itself an organisation split by tensions between professionalisers and others (White, 1985). Here a significant battle was fought in the 1990s over access to the occupation in the form of admission to membership for nursing assistants.

However, the trait theory of professions has more recently been seen to be unhelpful in understanding what professions are and how they work. As a theoretical underpinning for a profession-alising strategy, it has the difficulty that it is based on a false premise. Such traits may well define the characteristics of existing professions, such as medicine, but the suggestion that the pos-session of these characteristics was the primary cause of their attainment of professional status fails to acknowledge other poli-tical and economic imperatives. Sharpe and Faden (1998, p. 21), for example, suggest that 'the professional authority of physicians was consolidated in the mid-nineteenth century and early twentieth century ... both by chance and by design'. They link its develop-ment to the introduction of surgical antisepsis and diagnostic technologies, such as the stethoscope, as well as the growth in hospitals. The idea that another occupational group could attain the same status by adopting the characteristics of existing professions is thus called into question. However, a more important issue in the context of this discussion is that in so far as nursing attains these characteristics, it may well have to discard other values.

These traits are very much about control, and about inclusion and exclusion, and this has implications for other groups within society – notably patients. It can readily be suggested, for example, that the notion that only nursing can define the knowledge base and the portfolio of tasks to be undertaken serves to exclude other groups in society with legitimate interests. In their desire to exclude medicine from defining nursing, nurses may also effectively disenfranchise the general public and particular groups who might be assumed to have considerable relevant knowledge, such as people with dis-abilities, parents of small children, pregnant women, the elderly, and others. Interestingly this has given rise to a whole genre of nursing research which seeks to bring that knowledge, for example of the 'lived experience of disability', back into nursing.

The desire to control entry to the profession has led to a neglect of the kind of strategies for social inclusion that are increasingly commonplace in higher education and has created barriers to people, such as care assistants, with relevant skills and experience. The desire to 'distance' the occupation from everyday knowledge and skills is a means to engendering the sort of respect and awe which professions desire, but has a profoundly negative effect on society through privileging certain kinds of knowledge and experience over others. It also creates a distance between practitioner and client which inhibits communication and trust.

If we move beyond the trait theory we can find other ways of describing professions which also suggest that we should have concerns. For example, Hughes uses the concepts of *license* and *mandate* to describe professional activity in a way that helps us understand how it generates the potential for iatrogenic harm. Hughes (1971) defines these terms in the sociological classic, *The Sociological Eye*:

> 'An occupation consists in part in the implied or explicit *license* that some people claim and are given to carry our certain activities rather different from those of other people ... Generally ... they will also claim a *mandate* to define – not merely for themselves, but for others as well – proper conduct with respect to the matters concerned in their work. They will also seek to define ... modes of thinking and belief for everyone individually and for the body social and politic with respect to some broad areas of behaviour and thought.'
>
> Hughes (1971) cited in Walmsley *et al.*, 1993 p. 21

Hughes indicates that individuals within a profession are 'allowed' to do things which other people cannot and, importantly, they define what these things are. Doctors and dentists, for example, do things to patients which in another context would count as a very serious assault. They are not granted permission for this by the patient on the basis of an individual claim to knowledge or competence but because of their membership of a particular occupation which is presumed to 'own' a knowledge base that is not accessible to the general public. The case of Harold Shipman has been cited elsewhere in this book and we need to be clear that he was a serial killer and not an 'average' general practitioner. Nevertheless, the case is relevant here because his professional status served to legitimise his activities and to shield him from investigation both from inside or outside medicine. Clearly doctors, because of their professional status, are in a privileged position in which their actions are strongly assumed to be legitimate. Furthermore, they can dictate to the rest of us how we should think about a range of subjects, most obviously including illness and disease, surgery and other therapeutic interventions, but less obviously subjects such as pregnancy and childcare. The ability of the public legitimately to take a view different to that of medicine becomes eroded. This has perhaps been demonstrated most strongly in debates about the nature and management of childbirth, and in particular its locality.

## *Being a profession*

So, while it can be argued (by the professions) that the establishment of professions protects the public through internal self-regulation, it is apparent that there are also ways in which they can work against the interests of individuals and society. We can expand this debate by drawing briefly on critiques of professions from a number of fields. First, there is the critique of professions in general which has come from within sociology, and particularly those commentators who have looked at medicine and health care. Second, there are a number of commentators from within nursing who are unhappy about the potential consequences of profession-alising strategies. Third, and perhaps most useful of all, we can look at medicine as a comparative example and learn from their internal debates.

### A view from sociology

The critique of professions came from all sides of the ideological spectrum. The critique of Illich (1990) has been well described elsewhere in this book. It is based on the idea of a profession as disabling – as eroding the natural ability of individuals to manage their own lives. Similar critiques can be heard today in Britain and the USA suggesting that the welfare state has created a culture of dependency and eroded the self-sufficiency of individuals. In the 1980s Margaret Thatcher built on these critiques and mounted a substantial assault on the power of professions. However, critiques from other perspectives, including the political left, have suggested that professions create distance between health workers and clients; that professionals seek to control clients and that professionals tend to elevate the problem of their immediate client over the collective problems of the community. With specific reference to health care, key sociological commentators include Stacey (1992) who was also a lay member of the General Medical Council, and Davies (1995) who has looked at nursing regulation. They have particularly incorporated into the critique of profession the observation that the 'traditional' concept of profession is deeply gendered and integral to it are ideas about masculine activity and behaviour.

**A view from nursing**

Critical commentary has notably come from Salvage (1985) who argued, in the context of nursing, that professionalism:

- is divisive
- seeks to impose a uniform view
- denies the needs of its workers
- emphasises an individual approach
- does not challenge the status quo
- does not give strong support to the NHS.

This critique is also embedded in an approach to nursing which would want to see its value to society fully recognised and would in particular want to see the importance of its largely female work-force understood. This approach can also be seen in the writings of, for example, Robinson (1992) who was concerned that policies designed to support professionalisation, such as primary nursing, had profound and negative implications for the already margin-alised constituencies in the registered nursing workforce, such as black nurses (because they are more likely to be on different parts of the register) and nurses working part-time. Abbott and Meerabeau (1988) have also explored the implications of being professional. They comment, 'While the aim to be recognised as a professional occupation of equal status with medicine and the law may not yet have been achieved by nursing and social work, both occupations strive to differentiate themselves from the unqualified carer' (Abbot & Meerabeau, 1998 p. 10). The recognition that a profession should also value its workforce is becoming more apparent within medi-cine, but a tension remains between the professionalising policy of controlling entry and the proposal that in an unequal society and in recognition of the client constituency the ethical imperative should be towards the inclusion of otherwise marginalised and under-represented groups.

**A view from medicine**

Sir Donald Irvine, while President of the General Medical Council, the regulatory body for medicine, argued that '...professionalism in medicine rests on three pillars: expertise, ethics and service.... They are the basis of "professional autonomy"' (Irvine, 1999 p. 187). However, he went on to acknowledge that recent criticisms of the medical profession cast doubt on the strength of these pillars, although he was slightly ambiguous about whether this is a 'real' problem or a 'presentational' problem and therefore about whether the solution is a radical change of practice or a matter of reassurance of the public. He categorised the problems for the medical profession as follows:

- an unwillingness to demonstrate to the public that established doctors are competent
- allowing the impression that the profession does not protect the public from poor practice
- allowing a paternalistic attitude to pervade the profession
- allowing a conservative system of self-regulation
- a lack of openness and transparent accountability.

He indicated that these problems, if left unresolved, have the potential to erode the essential trust between the public and the profession which underpins self-regulation, and went on to show how the GMC and the profession is putting its house in order. However, the criticism of the medical profession is echoed by a number of other authors and a pervading theme is that at best the medical profession has not done much to help itself and, at worst, that the characteristics and values of the profession are inhibiting attempts to improve clinical practice. The criticism of the GMC, for example, is echoed by Walshe (1999 p. 7): 'The GMC has been much criticised for interpreting its mandate in a rather limited fashion. It has traditionally concerned itself largely with issues such as dishonesty, fraud, sexual misconduct and drug and alcohol abuse.' However, Walshe also includes the UKCC in his criticism, arguing that both the GMC and the UKCC had been largely reactive in their approach to maintaining standards of clinical practice.

Work on the actions and beliefs of individual practitioners reveals how these characteristics of the medical profession are manifested at an individual level. Rosenthal (1995, cited in Rosenthal, 1999 p. 150) quotes from her study of consultant attitudes: 'The moment you become a consultant in the UK, you are omni-competent. You don't have to pay attention to your colleagues; you don't have to pay attention to anyone.' Work by Vincent and Reason (1999) shows the consequences for junior doctors and other occupations; they describe a case in which the obstetric team – doctor and midwife – believed a Caesarean section was necessary but in which the consultant disagreed with the team and overrode their decision without giving due regard to their opinions. However, 'Both the midwife and the locum senior registrar were convinced of an obstruction, *but could not challenge the consultant*' (Vincent & Reason, 1999 p. 46, emphasis added). Eventually the senior nurse induced more evident signs of fetal distress (and considerable distress in the mother) in order to force a decision in favour of a Caesarean delivery.

A number of authors also refer to a climate in which most clinicians are reluctant to report matters of concern and in which there is a tacit norm of non-criticism (see Rosenthal, 1999, and Polywka & Chapman, 1999). Not only is it the case that practitioners cannot directly challenge the decision of colleagues, they feel unable to comment on or report the actions of other members of their profession. This problem lies behind some of Walshe's concerns about the reactive nature of the statutory regulatory bodies.

So, if we have evidence that the medical profession is not good at self-criticism or self-regulation, we might reasonably ask how it responds to attempts to regulate it from outside? Rosenthal's (1999) review of what we know about how doctors manage 'mishaps' provides some useful insights. She argues that the training to become a doctor provides them with a level of confidence in their ability to take decisions independently. Clinical practice is defined as individualistic rather than as a team endeavour. This results in a resistance to challenge from patients. Allsop and Mulcahy (1999) also looked at studies of how doctors responded to complaints from patients. They found that doctors were extremely upset by complaints because they believed them to be a challenge to their intrinsic self-worth – their status as doctors. Their view, as 'expert professionals' is that only their peers are qualified to comment on their actions – and as we have seen above this is an unlikely occurrence. Commentary from patients and relatives, or indeed managers, is therefore not regarded as a valid source of information and so cannot be the basis for an improvement strategy. It is important, however, to be clear that this does not mean that doctors do not take patient complaints seriously – they find them extremely challenging and difficult to deal with.

This brief commentary on the medical profession indicates that not only is medicine struggling to meet its own criteria for a profession: expertise, ethics and service, but also that doctors' training and modes of operating may be causing problems. That is to say, medicine does not have problems *despite* being a profession but in part *because* it is a profession. If nurses wanted to be professionals in the manner of doctors with the same structures and systems then they would become like doctors – and by the end of the twentieth century nobody wanted that. The issues were clear enough for Davies to comment in 1995: 'For nurses in the 1990s to look to professionalism, is thus to look to a model of practice that is under severe attack' (Davies, 1995 p. 137). This was not an entirely new idea. Oakley had commented a decade earlier 'The current crisis of confidence in medical care should tell us that professionalization is not the answer, that it may indeed be positively damaging to health' (Oakley, 1986 cited in Taylor & Field, 1993 p. 217). And Schön at about the same time had argued that, on the one hand, 'The professions have become essential to the very functioning of our society.' But on the other hand,

> '... there are increasing signs of a crisis of confidence in the professions. Not only have we witnessed well-publicised scandals in which highly esteemed professionals have misused their autonomy ... but we are also encountering visible failures of professional action. Professionally designed solutions to public problems have had unanticipated consequences, sometimes worse than the problems they were designed to solve.'
>
> Schön, 1983 p. 165

But they were not voicing a purely academic opinion – by 1995 a tide of general opinion was making itself heard, albeit still with difficulty until the more dramatic events of the late 1990s.

## A changing climate of opinion

These sociological and professional critiques have been powerfully reinforced by the national response to a number of incidents in which doctors were conclusively found to have acted against the interests of their patients. While these responses relate to particular incidents, it is clear that they connect to a broader spectrum of opinion which has more general concerns about the power of the medical profession and its lack of accountability. This has proved to be of considerable concern to the government – an indication of the importance of the medical profession to society – which has accepted the broader implications of the events at the Bristol Children's Hospital and produced a number of recommendations that relate to the training and practice of workers in the health care industry (DoH, 2002). By implication these are a critique of the activities of the professions in regulating themselves and represent new constraints on the power of the health care professions. It is possible to distinguish at least two elements in society's concerns. First, it can be said that the public has lost faith in the whole concept of professionalism. Professions (doctors and lawyers in particular) are increasingly seen as acting in their own interests rather than in the interests of the public. Second, and more specifically, the public has noticed that professions have been given special privileges on the basis of the assertion that they, and *only* they, could regulate themselves, but that the evidence that they are doing it is unconvincing.

## Options for the future

So, if adopting the mantle of a 'traditional' profession is neither a safe nor feasible option in the current climate, what strategies might be available to an occupation which wants to enhance its status and role in society but not at the expense of patient safety. One option is to eschew the pursuit of 'profession', admit that nursing is a trade wracked by internal divisions, and rely on good management to ensure patient safety. But what happens in the absence of professions? Would abolishing the professions – assuming that it could be done – solve the problem either of mistakes happening or of their being concealed? If professions do not self-regulate, then who does regulate health care practice? One obvious choice would be the client, but, within a state funded system of health care such as that of the UK, it is impossible to conceive that the state would simply stand back and allow individual consumers to dictate the shape and size of the health care system. A more likely candidate would be the state, and in relation to other occupations in the UK there is evidence that in the absence of a strong profession, the state rather than the consumer takes the major regulatory role. In school teaching, for example, we have seen increasing regulation through the imposition of the National Curriculum and through target setting for individual schools. Abbott and Meerabeau (1998) explore the problems of occupations employed by the state and without full professional status, particularly social work, and argue: 'Indeed, despite the current rhetoric of consumerism, problems are often defined by the state rather than the client, and workers are accountable to managers, not clients' (Abbott & Meerabeau, 1998 p. 10). The danger is that profession may be abandoned only in favour of bureaucracy. And the evidence from many child abuse enquiries does not demonstrate that the predominance of bureaucratic control any more than professional control ensures the safety of the client.

## A new sort of profession?

So, some sort of involvement of the profession in the management of clinical care standards seems desirable, but how can it best be managed? The critique of professions outlined above has been tempered by an evaluation of the benefits which they have brought to society – in some instances by the same commentator. Davies (1995) and Abbott and Meerabeau (1998) both quote Stacey (1992) in arguing for a 'new professionalism' which entails a re-evaluation of society's expectations of the professions. Stacey argues that professions could deliver better services if they reflected on their role in society. Stacey fully acknowledges that doctors have privileged their interests over those of their patients, in part through insisting on their exclusive rights to knowledge, expertise, and particularly status. However, 'she indicates that professions should build on the other nineteenth century ideal of service' (Abbott & Meerabeau, 1998 p. 7). She suggests that they must recognise the centrality of others, including patients, to health and healing, and accordingly adjust their idea of clinical autonomy, their control of the professions allied to medicine, and their claim to the exclusive right of the doctors to sit in judgment over other doctors. This new sort of 'reflective' profession would develop an understanding that, far from having a clear and unambiguous knowledge base, professions operate in a very complex and difficult environment in which there is considerable uncertainty and conflicting perspectives. Although medicine sought to manage uncertainty through building a hierarchical and defensive internal structure which excluded criticism (as discussed by Rosenthal *et al.*, 1999) – a strategy which is ultimately proving destructive – nursing could build a different structure through acknowledging the problem of uncertainty and developing shared responses with the client. Davies' new model profession 'involves a reflective practitioner who is engaged, embodied and creating an active problem-solving environment' (Davies, 1995 pp. 184–5).

In practice, a number of new frameworks for thinking about and developing the professional role have emerged, some driven directly by government while others have emerged from the professions themselves. What they have in common is an implicit emphasis on the management of risk in complex environments. The response of the state has been largely focused on organisational structures and processes. On the one hand it has embarked on what is termed 'modernising professions', which is essentially about changing the ways in which professions regulate themselves. At the same time, it has sought to incorporate the professions in the substantial infrastructure of quality assurance being created within the NHS at both the local and national level. In contrast, both medicine and nursing have generated internal movements which focused strongly on how individual practitioners fulfil their responsibilities, although their thinking has taken very different routes. Medicine has focused on evidence based practice, whereas nursing has developed reflective practice. Both have been taken up by government and incorporated into the national structures.

## The role of modern professions

Although the outward manifestation of clinical quality assurance is the creation of an organisational infrastructure of processes and committees, it was acknowledged that the overall aim of consistently delivering and enhancing quality could only be achieved through changing organisational culture. In effect, clinical governance (which is the term used for quality assurance structures in organisations involved in the delivery of health care) would work only by moving thinking away from the closed protectionism characterised by parts of the medical profession towards a more open culture in which mistakes could be discussed and learning encouraged. Clinical governance was never intended to work in isolation. On the one hand it needed to be supported by a national framework of standards and monitoring, and on the other it needed to create a dynamic interface with professional self-regulation. So, while managers have a key leadership role in relation to clinical governance, it is also the case that self-regulation, when properly done and properly accountable, is the most effective way of ensuring good practice (PHRU, 1998). It is the two working together that will, the present government (2002) believes, underpin quality improvement. This sentiment was echoed in 2002 by the Health Minister, John Hutton, who was reported in the *Times Higher Educational Supplement* (April 5, 2001) to have said that professional self-regulation underpins our aim to develop a modern, patient-centred NHS. Effective self-regulation reassures patients that the staff who treat them are fully qualified and trained in the most up-to-date practices.

A further manifestation of this belief comes in the expectations of the non-medical consultant posts. The document relating to the professions allied to medicine describes the role of senior practitioner in the NHS in the context of the new quality agenda. The requirements are many and onerous. It is clear that the consultant will act as an autonomous clinician much in the tradition of medical consultants exercising 'the highest degree of personal and professional autonomy, involving highly complex facts or situations, which require analysis and interpretation of data, leading to the implementation of a treatment or management strategy for the patient' (DoH, 2001b p. F9). However, it is also necessary for the consultant to create and develop protocols for care (for others to follow) and to provide 'expert input into the Trust's quality strategy, including influencing and delivering the clinical govern- ance agenda' (DoH, 2001b p. F9). The role of senior clinicians has been extended beyond the immediate delivery of care to their own clients to their collaboration with the managers and members of other occupational groups in the delivery of high quality care to all clients of the organisation. Furthermore, the same document makes it clear that they are also expected to actively identify and challenge organisational and professional barriers which inhibit service delivery.

As well as incorporating the professions more strongly into organisational structures, the state has also to change the way in which the health professions act by changing the national structures through which they are regulated. The aim is to both make them more efficient – and therefore more likely to be used – and more effective in defending the patient rather than the practitioner. Interestingly, the consultation document for the changes to the regulatory bodies defines the reactive nature of the proposals:

> 'It is clear from the Kennedy Report and the experience of pro- fessional regulation in recent years that there are weaknesses in the current arrangements which need to be addressed by reforms to the individual regulatory bodies, stronger and more effective co-ordination of their work and more robust accountability mechanisms.'
>
> DoH, 2001a p. 2

It also specified the driving forces for change: 'Modernisation [of professional regulation] must keep pace with change and devel- opment in the NHS as well as societal attitudes and public opinion' (DoH, 2001a p. 2). However, a tension between professional self- regulation and control and managerial responsibility for clinical governance remains; a tension well expressed in the title of a dis- cussion paper: *Clinical Governance, Striking a Balance Between Check- ing and Trusting* (Davies & Mannion, 1999). A key feature of the changes is the creation of a Council for the Regulation of Healthcare Professionals with the remit of protecting the interests of the public and which will work with the regulatory bodies for the professions to ensure a more integrated approach.

## Evidence based practice

Within the medical profession the development of evidence based practice was seen as a potential solution to reducing risk. Evidence based practice has been defined as 'an approach to decision making in which the clinician uses the best evidence available, in consultation with the patient, to decide upon the option which suits that patient best' (Gray, 1997 p. 9). It was developed in part because a number of doctors grew increasingly concerned with the lack of a good evidence base for clinical decisions – in the context of an occupation which claimed professional status in part on the grounds of having a secure and effective knowledge base, i.e. not commonsensical or experiential knowledge. A further spur to action was that doctors who knew that there was a good scientific evidence base for some decisions, found that it was not being used in everyday clinical decision making.

Traditionally, the 'evidence' on which medical practice has been based has been the natural science underpinnings, overlaid by the accumulated collective beliefs of the practitioners informed by research studies, often undertaken by pharmaceutical companies, overlaid again by the experience for the individual practitioner. In the evidence based practice movement of the 1990s (see, for example, Gray 1997) the concept of evidence was refined and deemed to refer specifically to 'hard' scientific evidence as produced largely, although not exclusively, through clinical trials. The problem was seen to be that each practitioner did not have the skills or the resources to evaluate the evidence properly. The solution was seen as training for practitioners, for example through the Critical Appraisal Skills for Practice programme (CASP), and the provision of 'pre-packaged' evaluations, such as those published in the journal *Bandolier*. The explicit rationale for *Bandolier* was that it would supply the bullets (of knowledge) to the practitioners (front line troops). It can be seen as an attempt to strengthen the profession's claim that its exclusive knowledge base was valid and that it therefore had the right to practise autonomously. The concept of evidence based practice has been increasingly incorporated into the government's strategies for change.

## Reflective practice

What can legitimately be called the reflective practice movement in nursing was developing just as the evidence based practice movement was enjoying growing success in medicine. Certainly nursing has become increasingly involved in evidence based practice, but for many nurses reflective practice has been a more accessible route to thinking about practice. In essence, reflective practice is just that, an injunction to reflect on and thereby learn from practice. The debates within reflective practice are largely about how, when and with whom this can best be achieved. Although the movement is based on the work of Schön (1983), who was originally analysing the work of architects, the development of reflective practice has come to seem special within nursing and to offer a unique way of thinking about health care practice. Certainly reflective practice offered nursing some relief from the difficulty of providing scientific evidence for the effectiveness of complex therapies and therapeutic processes which were hard to define and which were rarely under the complete control of nurses. More recently, the ideas of reflective practice have supported the development of clinical supervision – a system for enabling practitioners to reflect on their practice in a structured context which is intended to link practitioners to the management hierarchy in an open and supportive environment. In many ways this mirrors the ambition of clinical governance to promote a culture in which mistakes are acknowledged and used as the basis of learning, and some organisations have incorporated clinical supervision into their clinical governance processes. However, an important difference is that reflective practice remains based on the needs of the practitioner, whereas clinical governance focuses on the needs of the organisation – and of the patients.

## Conclusions

Salvage suggested as early as 1985 that we should no longer be asking hopefully 'Is nursing a profession?' but, 'Should nursing want to be a profession, and, if so, what do we mean by it?' (Salvage 1985, cited in Abbot and Meerabeau, 1998 p. 8). Medicine has, for a very long time, been taken to be a paradigm profession; which in practice was one which managed to be recognised as acting in the patients' best interests and thereby enhanced the standing of its members. And on that basis it was allowed to continue to regulate itself. However, recent events, which have cast doubt on the profession's concern for patients' rights and interests, and an increasing reluctance on the part of the public to practise deference to the members of established institutions of society, have led the government, the public, and increasingly the profession itself to question the training and motivation of practitioners and therefore the efficacy of existing arrangements for self-regulation. This is potentially bad news for nursing which has for many years aspired to the kind of autonomy, self-regulation and, most importantly status, enjoyed by medicine.

The establishment of the UKCC seemed at the time to be a

breakthrough which offered nursing some of the autonomy which medicine enjoyed and therefore the potential for parity of esteem and reward. Arguably this was always a chimera, given the unique historical context of medicine's progression to favoured profession, but in any case the 1990s were to see a substantial erosion in the public's confidence in professions in general. At a serious level there was increasing discussion of the failure of the social engineering of the 1960s (for example, the role of the architectural profession) and less seriously there was general contempt for the role of the new aspirant professions, such as estate agents, which operated without any visible service ethic. There have also been scandals outside medicine, such as the role of the auditors in the collapse of the Enron empire. However, medicine drew particular opprobrium, fuelled by a series of high profile scandals.

In the face of growing public disenchantment, and the consequent threat to a Labour government elected in part on its pledge to maintain and improve the performance of the NHS, the government chose a different approach to ensuring patient safety and the success of the NHS, one which embraces professionalism but only in a revised (and possibly etiolated) form. Because nursing has never been accepted as a full profession by the public it has escaped much of the contempt heaped on medicine in the wake of the Bristol enquiry. It is therefore well placed to participate fully in the new arrangements for quality put in place by the government. It is to be hoped that nursing can abandon the old agenda for professionalisation and embrace a 'new professionalism'. The question which it should be debating is whether the government's agenda for change is sufficient to ensure patient safety (as opposed to government safety) and is therefore deserving of support, or whether the profession should be pursuing a more radical agenda for change, perhaps in pursuance of Stacey's new ethic of public service and possibly one which acknowledges more forcibly the presence of the team in health care and indeed the central role of the client.

There is always a danger in a discussion such as this which focuses on the motivation and action of the practitioner(s), that the laity, both individually and collectively, are seen to be passive or at best reactive. However, recent events, such as the public's formidable responses to the 'official' pronouncements on CJD and BSE, show that the public in general is well able to discuss issues of risk and safety. Recent sociological commentary suggests that

> '...the structure of lay thought and perceptions of modern
> medicine is complex, subtle and sophisticated, and individuals

are not simply passive consumers who are duped by medical ideology. Rather they are critical reflexive agents who are active in the face of modern medicine and technological developments.'
Williams & Calnan, 1996 p. 1613

Indeed it could be said that if nurses are not ready to engage with the public on these issues, then they will become increasingly marginalised as agents of change in our society.

## *References*

Abbott, P. & Meerabeau, L. (eds) (1988) *The Sociology of the Caring Professions*, 2nd edn. UCL Press, London.

Allsop, J. & Mulcahy, L. (1999) Doctors' responses to patient complaints. In: *Medical Mishaps: Pieces of the puzzle* (eds M. M. Rosenthal, L. Mulcahy & S. Lloyd-Bostock), pp. 124–140. Open University Press, Buckingham.

Carpenter, M. (1977) The new managerialism and professionalism in nursing. In: *Classic Texts in Health Care* (eds L. Mackay, K. Soothill, & K. Melia) (1998), pp. 180–184. Butterworth Heinemann, Oxford.

Davies, C. (1995) *Gender and the Professional Predicament in Nursing*. Open University Press, Buckingham.

Davies, H. T. O. & Mannion, R. (1999) *Clinical Governance: Striking a balance between checking and trusting*. Centre for Health Economics, University of York, Discussion paper 165.

DoH (2001a) *Modernising Regulations in the Health Professions – Consultation Document*. Department of Health, London.

DoH (2001b) *Advance Letter PAM(PTA) 2/2001*. Department of Health, London.

DoH (2002) *Learning from Bristol: The Department of Health's Response to the Report of the Public Inquiry into Children's Heart Surgery at the Bristol Royal Infirmary 1984–1995*. The Stationery Office, London.

Gray, J. A. M. (1997) *Evidence-based Healthcare*. Churchill Livingstone, Edinburgh.

Hughes, E. C. (1971) *The Sociological Eye: Selected papers*. Aldine Atherton, Chicago.

Illich, I. (1990) *Limits to Medicine. Medical nemesis: the expropriation of health*. Penguin, London.

Irvine, D. (1999) Dysfunctional doctors: the General Medical Council's new approach. In: *Medical Mishaps: Pieces of the puzzle* (eds M. M. Rosenthal, L. Mulcahy & S. Lloyd-Bostock), pp. 185–196. Open University Press, Buckingham.

PHRU (1998) *Professional Self Regulation and Clinical Governance*. A report of a half day conference held at Regent's Park College Conference Centre, 13 October 1998. Public Health Resource Unit, Oxford pp. 26.

Polywka, S. & Chapman, E. J. (1999) Managing risk and claims: pieces of the puzzle. In: *Medical Mishaps: Pieces of the puzzle* (eds M. M. Rosenthal, L. Mulcahy & S. Lloyd-Bostock), pp. 221–227. Open University Press, Buckingham.

Robinson, K. (1992) The nursing workforce: aspects of inequality. In: *Policy Issues in Nursing* (eds J. Robinson, A. Gray & R. Elkan), pp. 24–37. Open University Press, Buckingham.

Rosenthal, M. M. (1999) How doctors think about medical mishaps. In: *Medical Mishaps: Pieces of the puzzle* (eds M. M. Rosenthal, L. Mulcahy & S. Lloyd-Bostock), pp. 141–153. Open University Press, Buckingham.

Rosenthal, M. M. Mulcahy, L. & Lloyd-Bostock, S. (eds) (1999) *Medical Mishaps: Pieces of the puzzle.* Open University Press, Buckingham.

Salvage, J. (1985) *The Politics of Nursing.* Heinemann Nursing, London.

Schön, D. A. (1983) The reflective practitioner: how professionals think in action. In: *Classic Texts in Health Care* (eds L. Mackay, K. Soothill, & K. Melia) (1998), pp. 164–170. Butterworth Heinemann, Oxford.

Sharpe, V. A. & Faden, A. I. (1998) *Medical Harm; Historical, Conceptual, Ethical Dimensions of Iatrogenic Illness.* Cambridge University Press, Cambridge.

Stacey, M. (1992) *Regulating British Medicine: The General Medical Council.* John Wiley, Chichester.

Taylor, S. & Field, D. (eds) (1993) *Sociology of Health and Health Care.* Blackwell Scientific Publications, Oxford.

Vincent, C. & Reason, J. (1999) Human factors approaches in medicine. In: *Medical Mishaps: Pieces of the Puzzle* (eds M. M. Rosenthal, L. Mulcahy & S. Lloyd-Bostock), pp. 39–56. Open University Press, Buckingham.

Walmsley, J. Reynolds, J. Shakespeare, P. & Woolfe, R. (1993) *Health, Welfare and Practice.* Sage, London.

Walshe, K. (1999) Medical accidents in the UK: a wasted opportunity for improvement. In: *Medical mishaps: Pieces of the puzzle* (eds M. M. Rosenthal, L. Mulcahy & S. Lloyd-Bostock), pp. 59–73. Open University Press, Buckingham.

Williams, S. J. & Calnan, M. (1996) The 'limits' of medicalization? Modern medicine and the lay populace in 'late' modernity. *Social Science and Medicine.* **42**, 1609–1620.

White, R. (1985) Political regulators in British Nursing. In: *Political Issues in Nursing: Past, present and future* (ed. R. White), pp. 19–45. John Wiley, Chichester.

# 4. *Harm Reduction in Context – The Scope of Nursing Practice*

*John Wilkinson and Joan P. McDowall*

## Introduction

In this chapter there is an exploration and discussion of evolving legislation, policy and professional regulation, all of which have been introduced to develop and coordinate the expanding scope of nursing practice. The context in which changes within nursing practice have emerged is described along with a critical commentary on the implications of these changes for public safety.

Within the United Kingdom there has been recent emphasis placed upon strategic moves from disease management towards health promotion (DoH, 1999a) with the establishment of expectations of the contributions to be made by nurses to this policy (DoH, 1999b). However, despite calls for nurses to change the way in which they operate, it has been claimed that nursing has traditionally lacked independence in the development of its own practice having been subject to a long history of political, managerial and medical control (Fatchett, 1998). If, as is claimed, nurses have historically been used as agents to serve the agendas of others, then the context within which nurses practise will sometimes be subject to influences which go beyond those which are solely directed to improvements in health care. In particular, there will always be a tension between the resources required to deliver good nursing care and the funding available to afford them. For example, consider the difficulties faced by nurses working in overstretched services, unsafe workplaces or when requested to implement treatment regimens which are contrary to the available evidence. These sorts of issues are clearly problematic for nurses as they can promote a dissonance between theory and practice, but they also have significant implications for the recipients of nursing care in that clinical judgement is subject to non-clinical constraints.

As well as being linked to financial resourcing, effective health care is essentially a very human activity which is dependent upon teamwork (DoH, 2000a). However, simply putting individuals or different groups together does not necessarily build strong team-working (Furnham, 1997). Effective teamwork comes about through sharing common goals and a collective understanding of the strategies to meet mutually agreed goals. Hence, nursing practice cannot be perceived in isolation from the activities of other providers of health care, the expectations of recipients of the care and the context within which health care is delivered. The challenge to nurses in the avoidance of iatrogenesis is the same as that facing all involved in health care: this is to be responsive when unnecessary harm through therapy occurs and, even more importantly, to be proactive in the prevention of such harm related to health care intervention. The key to changing well established ways of working is learning (Tiffany & Lutjens, 1998). All those who are involved in health care are expected to be life long learners (DoH, 2001a) both as individuals and as part of a learning culture (DoH, 2000a; 2001b). It is the purpose of this chapter to contribute to learning by outlining the context in which nursing practice is determined and highlighting some of the resulting consequences. It has been argued that a better understanding of the determinants and effects of nursing will inform more autonomous practice and this will lead to health care which is safer for the recipients of nursing care (Wilkinson, 1997).

## Nursing in the contemporary health care context

The expectation that NHS reforms will produce a more modern and dependable service call for an emphasis upon clinical governance to match previous requirements for corporate governance (DoH, 1997; 1998; 2000b). Clinical governance is about having an infrastructure to ensure consistently high clinical quality and the effective widespread dissemination of evidence based practice (Lugon & Secker-Walker, 1999). However, the UK government has acknowledged that the NHS still has much work to do in order to develop reliable processes to identify, analyse and systematically learn from lapses in standards of health care so that change can be strategically and promptly effected (DoH, 2001b).

Within nursing, a framework to universalise the best with regard to fundamental aspects of care has recently been launched in the form of clinical benchmarking (DoH, 2001c). Supported by a comprehensive toolkit and with a personal endorsement by the Chief Nurse of England, the clinical benchmarking initiative is a high profile strategy to critically evaluate key elements of care through processes of evidence review, reflection and comparison. Significantly there is strong emphasis upon patient, user and lay carer involvement in the determination of good nursing care. It is too early to analyse any effects of this project, but it is interesting to observe that attention to aspects of nursing deemed fundamental to nursing almost 150 years ago (Nightingale, 1859) still require extensive attention. Writing about Florence Nightingale, Skeet (1980) reflects upon the long established notion that while good nursing can make substantial contributions to health care, poor nursing can result in substantial unnecessary harm. In a context of rapid technological advances in health care, it is essential that nurses do not lose sight of the massive influence of basic core nursing skills upon health. A priority for nursing is to address concerns that core fundamental aspects of patient needs are, in some instances, not adequately addressed.

Whether health service reforms are in response to public concerns or whether media attention to the context in which these are occurring is a matter of opinion and it seems most likely that the media are reflecting as well as influencing that which is newsworthy. Whatever the trigger, health care is increasingly in the spotlight. Health care provider institutions are increasingly receiving intense and often critical media attention about service quality shortfalls. Individual practitioners have also attracted headlines for criminal acts (for example the murder convictions of Harold Shipman reported by Baker, 2001) and poor clinical practice (for example in the paediatric cardiothoracic surgical unit at Bristol Royal Infirmary reported by Kennedy *et al.*, 2000). It would seem that the general population have grounds to become increasingly sceptical of the benefits of entrusting themselves to professional health care.

An additional key factor, which may be influential upon public perceptions of health care, is the nature of health care need. It is accepted that many of the health needs within the United Kingdom are associated with chronic illness (DoH, 1999a). Indeed the national targets to reduce mortality due to cancer, heart disease, accidents and mental illness pose a substantial health promotion challenge to health care workers. This is because curative treatment is frequently restricted to situations where pathological harm is reversible (see Chapter 9), and hence much therapy is directed towards prevention of progressive deterioration or palliation. Within the scope of this text there are three important implications of providing a health service to a population which suffers substantial chronic illness which merit consideration.

i.   There are social responsibilities upon a society to ensure that there is fair access to information so that individuals and social groups are empowered to make healthy lifestyle decisions and so that they have access to the necessary resources to realise their choices. Nurses are expected to be proactive agents of health promotion (Forster, 2002) but to enable fulfilment of this role there are implications for nursing education and arrangements for service delivery, both of which require greater attention.

ii.  Clinical intervention for chronic illness is complex and frequently substantially invasive. Recent developments in pharmaceutical therapies are of particular relevance to nursing and are discussed in Chapter 5.

iii. Much chronic illness is longer term and this has ramifications for lifestyle and the adoption of coping strategies. There is a blurring of the distinction between health and illness as experience of a limiting long-standing illness becomes a normal way of life for the individual (Ong *et al.*, 1999). In this context the concept of the expert patient has emerged whereby health care professionals are encouraged to value the knowledge from experience of living with a chronic condition such as diabetes mellitus, depression or chronic obstructive pulmonary disease. Smith (2000) notes that this can be challenging for nurses who are used to being the experts themselves with a consequent expectation that patients should be passive recipients of their practice. Patient empowerment and partnership working will require an adjustment to working practices for many nurses and the teams in which they work.

A key message to emerge from the contemporary health care context is that there is a clear drive for quality health care services and safer outcomes from health care intervention. The mechanisms to achieve this are various, although two factors have achieved prominence. First, the government has sought to become more directive in how health care is delivered by setting out its strategy for clinical governance. Second, the public have increasing expectations of health care and a heightened awareness of the risks associated with health care delivery. Professional regulation within health care is undergoing a shift away from intra-professional investigation, that is peer review from within a discipline, towards greater accountability to public scrutiny. The remainder of this chapter will explore moves to make nurses more accountable to the government, their peers and, significantly, the public through an exploration of the arrangements for the regulation of nursing.

## *The professional regulation of nursing*

The professional regulation of nursing, until April 2002, was the function of the United Kingdom Central Council for Nursing, Midwifery and Health Visiting (UKCC) and the four National Boards for England, Northern Ireland, Scotland and Wales, all of which have now been replaced by the Nursing and Midwifery Council (NMC). A key aspect of the composition of the NMC is greater representation of the public in its membership. At the time of writing the precise details of how the NMC will function are not yet clear, but there has been close collaboration between the UKCC and the NMC and so it is expected that interim arrangements will be in place for a transition period until the new regulatory body begins to effect change on its own behalf. As the NMC (2002) will build upon the previous work of the UKCC and National Boards, the previous arrangements will be briefly outlined.

The primary function of nursing regulation is to protect the public. The achievement of this responsibility is through the maintenance of a register of qualified practitioners which is accessible to the public and employers, and to set standards and guidelines to regulate and guide practice. The professional register is a live register which means that all those admitted to it have had to demonstrate that they have been successful in completing, to an agreed standard, an appropriate programme of education at an approved institution. In order to remain on the register all registrants need to confirm every three years that they have engaged in continuing professional development to ensure the currency of their practical experience and theoretical knowledge and have recorded this lifelong learning in a professional portfolio of evidence of learning. Registrants also pay a fee to the regulatory council to enable it to fund its activities.

To regulate and guide practice, the UKCC made its standards and guidelines for professional nursing, health visiting and midwifery practice widely available. It was available to advise anyone with an enquiry about the professional activity of an individual nurse, or about issues related to the practice of nursing. The reference point for judging expectations of nurses are laid out in the UKCC Code of

Professional Conduct (UKCC, 1992) which is expanded upon in the guidelines for professional practice (UKCC, 1996). Pyne (1998) argues that the introduction of the Code of Professional Conduct was significant because its intention was to encourage nurses to think of their practice as dynamic, being subject to changing needs and development through learning. The intention of the code is to provide clear principles with which practice must comply, but not to be interpreted in a way which is limiting or restrictive. One of the UKCC's final acts was to consult upon and agree a revised set of professional standards which were endorsed by both the UKCC and the NMC at a joint meeting.

As the scope of practice continues to expand, nurses are required to exercise sound judgement by drawing upon diverse sources of information to inform professional decision making. Each nurse is accountable for his or her professional actions. In forming decisions about practice a nurse is expected to consider very carefully the Code of Professional Conduct, the quality of available evidence, local policies, the law and his or her critical reflections upon previous experiences. A key obligation is for every nurse to be fully aware of his or her professional boundaries and personal limitations and to work within these by declining to undertake responsibilities for which they are not competent or which are contradicted by the Code of Professional Conduct.

Working within personal capabilities can give rise to tensions within practice. Consider a situation where a patient asks for care which falls outside a particular nurse's personal framework of competent practice: for example, a request by an elderly man to remove ear wax by syringing. In this case it would be appropriate for the nurse to explain that he or she was not able to perform the procedure and to make arrangements for the patient to be assessed by someone appropriately skilled in the management of this condition. The patient may not understand why his request is not met by the nurse and complain that 'everyone else does it'. It is important that the nurse is not persuaded to proceed as he or she is the judge of professional competence, not the patient. Referral to a competent colleague is a responsible course of action which avoids putting the patient at risk of harm, ensures that the patient is assessed for the care to meet his or her needs and prevents the nurse from working outside his or her field of competency. It may be that the nurse's manager expresses surprise that the nurse is unable to perform the ear syringing and an instruction is given to 'get on with it – it's part of your job'. Again, assertiveness is required on the part of the nurse to insist that this aspect of care is inappropriate given an awareness of personal practice boundaries. The nurse would not be able to transfer professional accountability to someone else such as a manager. It is also unacceptable for someone else to assume accountability for another, hence for example, a doctor who said 'don't worry, do it and I'll cover you' is not acceptable as the nurse concerned would not be working within his or her scope of professional practice. Personal actions or omissions cannot expect to be excused by claiming to act on the instructions of another person. If ear syringing is likely to be a commonly encountered aspect of practice, then it would be reasonable for the manager to work with the nurse to ensure that appropriate steps are taken to enable him or her to develop the relevant competence to meet similar patient needs in future. Through negotiation, learning and supervision the nurse is thus able to develop his or her practice to respond to patients' needs safely.

If a nurse is thought to have practised outside of the Code of Professional Conduct, then anyone (for example a patient, relative, colleague or employer) can report their concerns to the regulatory body. In practice, such a referral is usually after a local investigation has taken place in the workplace, commonly in the form of implementing a disciplinary policy. It should be noted that the function of a nursing regulatory council is to protect the public through the application of professional standards and hence is restricted to the consideration of issues which are related to professional registration. Locally unresolved issues relating to contracts of employment which do not involve concerns about professional standards are dealt with by implementing local policies, the Arbitration, Conciliation and Advisory Service (ACAS) or at an employment tribunal (Willey, 2000).

Details of how the UKCC responded to complaints about professional conduct were produced in a clear format (UKCC, 1998) so that access to the process was readily available. Initially referrals to the UKCC were considered at a Preliminary Proceedings Committee (PPC). The PPC initiated any investigations and collected any evidence it deemed necessary to make a judgment on the case before them. If there were concerns about the protection of the public from further risks, then the PPC could order a suspension from practice pending the outcome of investigations and any subsequent action by the UKCC. At the end of an investigation by the PPC there are a number of possible outcomes:

- a decision not to proceed any further and to consider the matter closed as there is no cause for concern

- to decide to carry out further investigations
- to consider the appropriateness of issuing a caution to the registrant
- to refer the matter to the Health Committee of the UKCC to consider health related fitness to practice or
- to refer the matter to the Professional Conduct Committee (PCC) of the UKCC to consider conduct related fitness to practice.

Where an investigation by the PPC found that there was evidence of misconduct by a nurse, he or she would be notified of the allegation and the decision to refer the matter to the PCC. The PCC would invite the registrant, and a representative if desired, to its proceedings which are held in public. At the committee hearing the UKCC would present any relevant evidence and witnesses as would the registrant. At the end of a hearing before the PCC there were a number of possible outcomes:

- postponement of judgment pending more evidence
- no action
- the issue of a caution
- referral to the Health Committee of the UKCC
- suspension from the register for a specified period or
- removal from the register.

Applications for restoration to the register are received and these are considered in the light of the reasons for original removal and any remedial activity engaged in by the former registrant.

The UKCC therefore discharged its duty to protect the public using the PPC and PCC as necessary. It is expected that the NMC will function along similar lines, and the details of its arrangements will emerge in due course. The challenge to the NMC is to build upon the work of the UKCC, but to do so in a way that reflects the contemporary health care context already highlighted. As such, the NMC will need to satisfy an increasingly critical population who are demanding assurances of public protection from incompetent health care providers.

An important aspect of professional regulation is to fulfil public protection responsibilities while at the same time ensuring fairness of consistency to registrants in the way that they are investigated and dealt with when professional misconduct allegations arise. Professional practice occurs within a complex milieu and it is essential that any investigation into misconduct reflects the context in which it takes place. When breaches of the Code of Professional

Conduct are considered by the regulatory council it is important that these are viewed holistically. Dimond (2002a) cites the case of a community psychiatric nurse who was considered by the UKCC for not maintaining up-to-date records on the patients under his care. This particular example shows that although there was no question that several clauses of the Code of Professional Conduct were breached, the UKCC was able to consider mitigating circumstances and the fact that the registrant had learnt from his misconduct. In this instance the UKCC issued a caution rather than removed the nurse from the register.

It should be noted that public protection responsibilities extend to nurses themselves who are acknowledged to count as members of the public as well as having obligations to adhere to professional standards. Dimond (2002b) reports a case of the UKCC taking action over a male charge nurse who was guilty of sexually harassing female nursing subordinates. This particular case is important because it gives a clear message that misconduct and unnecessary harm to colleagues is as significant as that suffered by patients, clients or their associates.

## Accountability of nurses beyond professional regulation

As well as being subject to their own professional regulatory arrangements nurses are therefore also members of the public themselves and, in most circumstances, employees of a health providing organisation. In both of these latter guises there are legal obligations which are in place to ensure protection of patients, but which also serve to safeguard the rights of other relevant parties such as nurses themselves, colleagues with whom they work and their employers.

As members of the public, nurses are subject to the law. Legal issues which are specifically relevant to nurses are considered in detail by Dimond (1995) who explains that nurses are accountable under all aspects of the law and, if they break it, can expect to face the consequences of their actions. Hence, patients, relatives and colleagues are protected against criminal acts against them by nurses (for example theft, assault) or civil wrongs (for example negligence, breaches of confidentiality). The courts have the authority to judge if a nurse is guilty of a criminal offence and impose an appropriate sentence or, if a nurse is liable for a civil wrong, to order the payment of compensation. Importantly, Caulfield (2002) makes the point that the legal and professional responsibilities of nurses are separate and as such are dealt with separately. Only the NMC has the power to determine whether a nurse has breached the Professional Code of Conduct and to prohibit the entitlement to work as a nurse. A court or any other person involved in a nurse's misdemeanour may approach the NMC with their concerns about the professional behaviour of a nurse. As already outlined, the UKCC had processes to undertake its own investigation and decide subsequent courses of action and this will continue under the new arrangements to be brought in by the NMC.

If a nurse is an employee of a health providing organisation then he or she is protected under, and obliged to work within, employment law. Effective and harmonious working arrangements are dependent upon a culture of partnership between employers and employees (Willey, 2000). This is of particular relevance in the area of employment law which regulates health and safety at work where accountability for safety is a dual responsibility held by both employers and employees (Health and Safety Commission, 1998). In a health care work setting, responsibilities for safety naturally include patients and their visitors. In addition to proactive measures to ensure a safe working environment and the provision of safe equipment such as moving and handling apparatus, it is important for individuals and organisations to be reactive to unsafe occurrences and near misses. Thus, the reporting of accidents and adverse events, analysis of trends, the formulation of action plans and evaluation of action taken are key aspects of good safety management. Nurses must therefore ensure that they have the necessary assertiveness skills in order to come forward and report actual and potential safety incidents. In turn managers must take steps to set up streamlined systems for the processing and actioning of issues that are brought to their attention.

## The dynamic and expanding role of nursing

The changing and complex nature of health care has already been highlighted earlier in this chapter. In response to these developments, nursing theory and practice have become more diverse and increasingly complicated. At the same time, changes in post-graduate medical education and working time regulations have resulted in a reduction in the duration of duty rosters for junior doctors (NHSME, 1992; Wilkinson & Wilkinson, 1995) with consequential effects upon the substitution of nurses into roles previously undertaken by doctors. This trend is continuing in nursing role development as part of the NHS Plan (DoH, 2000b). A systematic review of randomised control trials and observational research on nurse practitioners in primary care concluded that increasing the availability of them is likely to lead to high levels of patient satisfaction and high quality care (Horrocks *et al.*, 2002). Furthermore, the British Medical Association (BMA, 2002) has recently proposed a model of primary health care in a discussion document in which nurses take on much greater levels of responsibility and autonomy as part of an integrated team. This has been received with mixed responses from influential figures within nursing. Beverley Malone, General Secretary of the Royal College of Nursing, has commented that '...the RCN has long argued that nurses are competent to deal with the wide range of illnesses and minor injuries that patients have' (*RCN Bulletin*, 2002, p. 1). However, while voicing some cautious support, Helen Scott, editor of the *British Journal of Nursing*, contrastingly also says that '...the nursing profession needs a period of consolidation before it decides to change the boundaries of its practice' (Scott, 2002, p. 296). The dynamic and expanding role of nursing is clearly the topic of discussion and controversy from a professional perspective and this debate must include consideration of the strengths and limitations of change for patients.

Walsh (2000) delineates between two aspects of the developing roles within nursing termed the *extended role* and the *expanded scope* of practice. Extended roles refer to clearly identified tasks, often technical in nature, such as venepuncture, intravenous cannulation and suturing of wounds. Since the 1970s many nurses have taken on such roles after a period of training and assessment leading to certification. As most of such tasks were formerly the exclusive domain of doctors, much of the responsibility for teaching and assessment fell to doctors. This system is underpinned by the assumption that the medical staff involved were competent at the task themselves, and that they were able to teach and assess appropriately. Humphris and Masterson (2000) argue that the requirement for nurses to obtain certificates of competence for extension to their role has perpetuated a culture of nursing subservience to medical dominance. Nurses who are able to undertake additional roles can become in demand within a hospital or community care setting to move from patient to patient to perform their skills. This in turn requires other nurses to undertake the remaining aspects of nursing care which has the effect of breaking nursing work down into a series of delegated tasks and the consequential outcome of fragmented care for individual patients. This puts great pressure on effective communication relating to care planning and record keeping in order to achieve continuity of care. Panel 4.1

**Panel 4.1**   Fragmented care and poor communication.

> A man was admitted to hospital for an arthroscopy on his knee. He
> had a history of thrombosis which he reported to the nurse practitioner
> on admission who recorded the information in his assessment docu-
> mentation. A different nurse who worked on the day surgery ward
> completed the patient's pre-operative documentation and did not
> indicate the thrombosis risk on the form. The operation was carried out
> and the patient was discharged from hospital the same day. Two days
> later the man was admitted to the intensive care unit of another hos-
> pital with a pulmonary embolus which might have been prevented by
> anti-coagulant drugs and appropriate discharge advice.
>
> (Adapted from Department of Health, 2000a)

illustrates the problems which may arise in relation to fragmented
care and poor communication between those providing care.

The term expanded scope of practice refers to the development of
nursing roles which can be employed within a repertoire of nursing
practice for the benefit of patient-centred care (Castledine & McGee,
1998). Some of the same tasks associated with an extended role may
be relevant, but the difference is that these are incorporated into
nursing practice as part of a sequence of care delivered by a nurse.
Panel 4.2 outlines an example of how a nurse with an expanded
scope of practice can enhance patient care.

Consider an alternative to the situation described in Panel 4.2.
The patient would have to wait until a doctor or nurse who had the
skills to perform the re-cannulation was free, but who perhaps was
not familiar with either the patient or his particular clinical or
personal needs. Precious human resources must be managed
responsibly and to maximum patient benefit and it may be attractive for managers to allocate staff duties in a way that matches
specific skills to particular patient needs. Indeed, it is arguable that
allocations to specific tasks and adherence to routine can be useful
to reducing error as such approaches are designed to avoid omission of safety checks. However, attempts to deliver health care in a
conveyor belt assembly line fashion can be impersonal and must be
avoided. Paul Barber, a nurse himself, reports his own experiences
as a patient (Barber, 1997). Barber's experiences offer insights for
nurses which suggest that avoidable harm can occur if nursing
health care is not sufficiently patient centred. Safe practice is
dependent upon task ability which should be informed by specific
patient needs and which is inclusive of relevant knowledge, skills
and attitudes, not any aspect in isolation. An example of unsafe

**Panel 4.2** An example of a nurse with an expanded scope of practice enhancing patient care.

Mary Smith is a registered nurse working on a surgical ward in a general hospital. She has attended a course in venepuncture which was developed by a practice development nurse (PDN) who works within her directorate. Following the course Mary received guidance on the practical aspects of venepuncture from her PDN and her clinical nurse leader (CNL) who is her named mentor. Mary became confident of her skills in venepuncture under supervision based upon her understanding of the principles of fluid management in surgical patients and she asked her CNL to assess her competence. Following agreement of competence between Mary and her CNL Mary felt confident that she could exercise her judgement on when she might add venepuncture to her repertoire of practice.

A few days later Mary was on duty when a patient under her care reported a painful cannula insertion site which was in situ to enable an intravenous infusion of crystalloid solution. Mary assessed the cannula as having tissued. Mary was aware of the hydration needs of her patient and the current status of his fluid balance. She was also aware of the patient's drug regimen which included prescriptions for intravenous drugs. The patient had been complaining of feeling grubby and had mentioned how he would like to take a bath and change his clothes. Mary was able to discontinue the infusion, which enabled the patient to attend to his hygiene needs independently with less inconvenience due to removal of the infusion. The original line was inserted in theatre in the left hand, but Mary re-sited the cannula in the right hand as she was aware that her patient was left handed. The intravenous therapy was recommenced within a timeframe which did not compromise the appropriate delivery of drugs and fluids by this route.

delineation of role according to task allocation is presented in Panel 4.3.

The NHS Plan (DoH, 2000b) gives ten examples of how nurses might expand their practice in areas as diverse as managing a case load, prescribing, advanced life support and judging the need for ordering clinical investigations. The challenge to nursing in meeting these targets is to avoid the potential and actual consequences of fragmentation of nursing care through the development of therapeutic relationships with each of their patients so that they are cared for in the context of their individual needs.

Working in a patient-centred way should be the goal of everyone involved in health care. Nurses will have to work in collaboration with other disciplines within the health service, but also across the

**Panel 4.3** Unsafe task allocation, an example of patient observation when administering a blood transfusion.

It is possible to learn how to observe and record basic clinical observations (temperature, pulse, respiration and blood pressure) relatively quickly and hence this is a task which might be readily delegated to an inexperienced member of a care team. However, it has been well established by research into blood transfusion errors (Linden *et al.*, 1992; Tourault & Mummert, 1994) that poor recognition of adverse reactions and lack of appropriate action is not uncommon and this has led to fatal consequences. In a review of the literature in this area Wilkinson & Wilkinson (2001) found that sometimes patient deterioration due to a suspected haemolytic reaction was well documented, but that there was no reporting of findings nor intervention undertaken and the transfusion was allowed to continue.

In these cases it would appear that the practitioner who undertook the clinical observations was skilled in that particular task, but patients came to harm because nursing staff lacked the relevant competencies in making interpretations of their findings and were unaware of the appropriate action they should take, even if this was limited to referral for assistance. Task competency was insufficient to ensure patient safety because it was not integrated within a repertoire of patient care.

entire social care sector. Local strategic partnerships (Department of the Environment, Transport and the Regions, 2001) are a government initiative to encourage community strategies which develop partnerships between public services in the key target areas of education, employment, crime, health and housing. Clearly these are all interrelated and are highly relevant to the quality of life within a local community. The intention is to integrate services and to avoid the problems of omission, replication, fragmentation and contradiction which are frequently associated with separate services that operate in isolation from each other. To make a legitimate contribution to new ways of delivering public services, nursing leaders and individual practitioners need to develop effective lines of communication with other community agencies and develop roles flexibly to meet care needs. A failure of nursing to embrace an approach to meeting health care needs which integrates services will not serve the health needs of a community and the individuals in it.

If nursing is to develop as a workforce in order to be responsive to changing health care delivery contexts, there will be widespread implications for nursing education to develop skills in the facilitation of flexible learning. This has already been commenced with a substantial revision of entry to register education (UKCC, 1999) which introduced renewed emphases upon wider concepts of health and a refocus upon clinical skills. Attention has recently been directed to continuing professional development for health care professionals in general (DoH, 2001a) and nurses in particular (ENB/DoH, 2001). Evidence of continuing professional development is a well established obligation of remaining on the professional register, and it seems likely that the NMC will seek to strengthen expectations within this requirement. Evidence of lifelong learning is central to ensuring patient safety in the inevitable dynamic and expanding role of nursing and the challenge to workforce development confederations, and nursing education, is to develop ways that this can be facilitated in an effective and flexible manner.

## Conclusion

In this chapter there has been an outline of the contemporary health context with attention drawn to the implications for nursing, particularly in relation to patients' safety. The role of professional regulation in protecting the interests of the public has been considered at a time when this is undergoing considerable adjustment related to the establishment of the Nursing and Midwifery Council (NMC). A particular challenge to the NMC will be to fulfil its obligations to public safety through professional standards at a time of rapid change particularly relating to the dynamic and expanding role of nursing.

Although changes in health care provision and nursing practice are designed to enhance patient care, it has been shown that this can also be associated with risks to patient safety. The central purpose of professional regulation is to protect the public, but current levels of adverse events suggest that there is more to be done proactively to prepare nurses for the roles facing them and to support and guide them in the course of their practice. This is work which will require collaboration within nursing, drawing upon contributions from individual practitioners, nursing leaders, nursing academics, professional organisations and the NMC. In the development of nursing, nurses will also need to work in close partnership with key stakeholders such as patient and user representative forums, employers and managers, trade unions, politicians and government. It is clear that the key to public safety is professional education, support and guidance and not simply the fear of professional regulatory mechanisms which, although essential, are a symptom of the failure of the former.

# *References*

Barber, P. (1997) Caring – the nature of a therapeutic relationship. In: *Nursing: A knowledge base for practice* (ed. A. Perry), pp. 230–271, 2nd edn. Edward Arnold, London.

Baker, R. (2001) *Harold Shipman's Clinical Practice, 1974–1998.* Department of Health, London.

BMA (2002) *The Future Healthcare Workforce.* British Medical Association, London.

Castledine, G. & McGee, P. (eds) (1998) *Advanced and Specialist Nursing Practice.* Blackwell Science, Oxford.

Caulfield, H. (2002) Legal issues. In: *Common Foundation Studies in Nursing* (eds N. Kenworthy, G. Snowley & C. Gilling), pp. 113–129, 3rd edn. Churchill Livingstone, Edinburgh.

Department of the Environment, Transport and the Regions (2001) *Local Strategic Partnerships.* The Stationery Office, Norwich.

Dimond, B. (1995) *Legal Aspects of Nursing*, 2nd edn. Prentice Hall, London.

Dimond, B. (2002a) Psychiatric nurse who was too busy to keep up-to-date records. *British Journal of Nursing.* **11**, 226.

Dimond, B. (2002b) Sexual harassment of female nursing students. *British Journal of Nursing.* **11**, 300.

DoH (1997) *The New NHS: Modern, dependable.* The Stationery Office, London.

DoH (1998) *A First Class Service.* The Stationery Office, London.

DoH (1999a) *Saving Lives: Our healthier nation.* The Stationery Office, London.

DoH (1999b) *Making a Difference: Strengthening the nursing, midwifery and health visiting contribution to health and health care.* The Stationery Office, London.

DoH (2000a) *An Organisation with a Memory.* The Stationery Office, London.

DoH (2000b) *The NHS Plan.* The Stationery Office, London.

DoH (2001a) *Working Together, Learning Together.* The Stationery Office, London.

DoH (2001b) *Building a Safer NHS for Patients.* The Stationery Office, London.

DoH (2001c) *Elements of Care.* The Stationery Office, London.

ENB/DoH (2001) *Preparation of mentors and teachers.* English National Board/Department of Health, London.

Fatchett, A. (1998) *Nursing in the New NHS: Modern, dependable?* Ballière Tindall, London.

Forster, D. (2002) The nurse as a health promoter. In: *Common Foundation Studies in Nursing* (eds N. Kenworthy, G. Snowley & C. Gilling), pp. 279–309, 3rd edn. Churchill Livingstone, Edinburgh.

Furnham, A. (1997) *The Psychology of Behaviour at Work.* The Psychology Press, Hove.

Health and Safety Commission (1998) *Safety Representatives and Safety Committees.* 3rd edn. The Stationery Office, Norwich.

Horrocks, S., Anderson, E. & Salisbury, C. (2002) Systematic review of whether nurse practitioners working in primary care can provide equivalent care to doctors. *British Medical Journal.* **324**, 819–823.

Humphris, D. & Masterson, A. (2000) *Developing New Clinical Roles.* Churchill Livingstone, London.

Kennedy, I., Howard, R., Jarman, B. & McLean, M. (2000) *The Inquiry into the Management of Care of Children Receiving Complex Heart Surgery at the Bristol Royal Infirmary. Interim Report – Removal and Retention of Human Material.* The Bristol Royal Infirmary, Bristol.

Linden, J., Paul, B. & Dressler, K. (1992) A report of 104 transfusion errors in New York State. *Transfusion.* **32**, 601–606.

Lugon, M. & Secker-Walker, J. (eds) (1999) *Clinical Governance: Making it happen.* Royal Society of Medicine Press, London.

NHSME (1992) *Junior Doctors: The new deal.* National Health Service Management Executive, London.

Nightingale, F. (1859) *Notes on Nursing.* Churchill Livingstone, Edinburgh, reprinted 1980.

Nursing & Midwifery Council (2002) Nursing & Midwifery Council: Your new regulatory body. *N&MC News.* NMC, London.

Ong, B., Jordan, K., Richardson, J. & Croft, P. (1999) Short report: experiencing limiting long-standing illness. *Health and Social Care in the Community.* **7**, (1) 61–68.

Pyne, R. (1998) *Professional Discipline in Nursing, Midwifery and Health Visiting,* 3rd edn. Blackwell Science, Oxford.

Royal College of Nursing Bulletin (2002) *RCN welcomes BMA Discussion Paper.* RCN, Harrow.

Scott, H. (2002) BMA proposes radical changes to the nursing role (Editorial). *British Journal of Nursing.* **11**, 296.

Skeet, M. (1980) *Notes on Nursing.* Churchill Livingstone, Edinburgh.

Smith, U. (2000) Top 10 tips for working with expert patients. *Nursing Times.* **96**, (26) 29.

Tourault, M. & Mummert, T. (1994) Transfusion related fatality reports – a summary. *Nurse Management.* **25**, (10) 80I, 80L, 80O.

Tiffany, C. & Lutjens, L. (1998) *Planned Change Theories for Nursing.* Sage, London.

UKCC (1992) *Code of Professional Conduct,* 3rd edn. United Kingdom Central Council for Nursing, Midwifery & Health Visiting, London.

UKCC (1996) *Guidelines for Professional Practice,* 3rd edn. United Kingdom Central Council for Nursing, Midwifery & Health Visiting, London.

UKCC (1998) *Complaints about Professional Conduct.* United Kingdom Central Council for Nursing, Midwifery & Health Visiting, London.

UKCC (1999) *Fitness for Practice.* United Kingdom Central Council for Nursing, Midwifery & Health Visiting, London.

Walsh, M. (2000) *Nursing Frontiers, Accountability and Boundaries of Care.* Butterworth Heinneman, Oxford.

Wilkinson, C. & Wilkinson, J. (1995) What are the implications of doctor–nurse substitution? (Editorial). *British Journal of Nursing.* **4**, 855.

Wilkinson, J. (1997) Developing a concept analysis of autonomy in nursing practice. *British Journal of Nursing.* **6**, 703–707.

Wilkinson, J. & Wilkinson, C. (2001) Administration of blood transfusions to adults in general hospital settings: a review of the literature. *Journal of Clinical Nursing.* **10**, 161–170.

Willey, B. (2000) *Employment Law in Context.* Pearson Education Limited, Harlow.

# 5. Expanding Nurse Prescribing and the Hidden Harm within Modern Drug Therapy

*Jennifer Kelly*

'There are some patients whom we cannot help: there are none whom we cannot harm.'

Arthur M. Bloomfield MD, quoted in Lambert (1978)

## Introduction

Drugs are used as the panacea for many of our problems. We take them when we are ill for diagnostic and therapeutic purposes and we take them when we are healthy as prophylaxis, as well as for social and recreational purposes. This dependence on drugs is a major cause of iatrogenic harm, for every drug that has the potential to do us good also has the potential to do us injury, especially when one appreciates that the only difference between a drug and a poison is the dose. From a medical perspective, drugs can be defined as chemical substances which are used in the prevention or treatment of a disease with the intention of improving the patient's condition. They range from caffeine and vitamins through to narcotics and cytotoxic chemotherapy, and most of them are derived from plants. Many of these plants, e.g. digoxin, curare, have undergone critical clinical assessment and been accepted into orthodox medicine, often as the isolated and chemically standardised active ingredient (D'Arcy, 1991).

This chapter will look at the iatrogenic harm that drugs can cause. It will consider adverse reactions to orthodox drugs, before exploring the problems of herbal remedies, which many people are now turning to as they become disillusioned with conventional drug therapy. The chapter will then go on to consider the issue of non-compliance, on the part of both patients and health care staff, and how it can lead to harm, including drug errors, which will be addressed in some detail. Finally, the chapter will address the issue of nurse prescribing and its potential for increasing iatrogenic harm if it is not implemented carefully.

## Adverse drug reactions – what are they, and can they be prevented?

The iatrogenic potential of drugs is demonstrated by the fact that nearly 10,000 people a year in the UK are reported through the yellow card system organised by the Committee on Safety of Medicines and the Medicines Control agency to have experienced serious adverse reactions to drugs (DoH, 2000a). A meta-analysis of 39 prospective studies carried out in the United States over a period of 32 years identified that the overall incidence of adverse reactions is 6.7%, and that of fatal adverse reactions is 0.32% of hospitalised patients (Lazarou *et al.*, 1998). Thus in the USA in 1994, 2,216,000 hospitalised patients had serious adverse drug reactions, whilst in 106,000 patients the effects were fatal, making adverse drug reactions around the fourth leading cause of death in hospital. However, a study by Jha *et al.* (1998) suggests that the incidence of adverse drug events may be much higher than previously reported, as the methods used to collect the data affect the number and type of adverse reactions identified. Adverse drug reactions are defined by the World Health Organisation (WHO, 1966) as any noxious, unintended and undesired effect of a drug which occurs at doses used in humans for prophylaxis, diagnosis or therapy. These reactions can be classified in a number of ways, and Table 5.1 gives examples.

As can be seen from Table 5.1, adverse drug reactions are very variable. Some, like the Type A or augmented effects are predictable, as they are a characteristic of the drug. Thus for example, morphine is an effective painkiller because it binds to opioid receptors in the central nervous system and inhibits the passage of painful nervous impulses. However, the receptors to which it binds are also found in the gut where binding causes constipation. Thus, constipation is an expected side effect of opiate use and in severe cases of diarrhoea this side effect is used as a treatment for this condition. Although side effects are predictable, preventing them can be difficult. Reduction in the dose of drug administered is one method. The smallest effective dose should always be given, and then if need be the dose gradually increased to maximise the therapeutic effect. The oral contraceptive pill illustrates the positive benefits of reducing the dosage of a drug.

**Table 5.1**  Classification of adverse drug effects (Page *et al.*, 1997).

| Group | Definition | Examples |
|---|---|---|
| Augmented effects | Unwanted effects that occur as a result of the pharmacology of the drug. Includes side effects, secondary effects, drug interactions and toxicity effects. Relatively common and usually minor. | Hypotension due to anti-hypertensives. Opportunistic infections that may develop after antibiotic treatment. Interaction between aspirin and warfarin leading to haemorrhage. Anticoagulant induced haemorrhage. |
| Bizarre effects | Unpredictable unwanted effects that are not dose-related. Relatively uncommon, but they have a high rate of morbidity and mortality. Includes intolerance, idiosyncrasy, and allergic or hypersensitivity reactions. | Intolerance to lactose – used to give bulk to medicines. Hyperpyrexia due to halothane. Anaphylaxis due to penicillin. |
| Chronic effects | Unwanted effects that occur after prolonged treatment. | Phenothiazine-induced Parkinsonism. Colonic dysfunction from laxative abuse. |
| Delayed effects | Unwanted effects that do not occur for years after treatment has started and/or finished. May affect the next generation. | Secondary cancers after treatment with cytotoxic chemotherapy. Carcinoma of the vagina in daughters of women who took diethylstilbestrol (stilboestrol) during pregnancy. |
| End of use effects | Withdrawal effects, i.e. unwanted effects that occur when the drug is suddenly stopped. | Adrenocortical insufficiency after stoppage of glucocorticoids. Delirium tremens when stopping drinking alcohol. |

Here a reduction in drug dosage since the early 1980s has minimised the risk of deep vein thrombosis whilst maintaining good levels of protection against pregnancy.

A second possible way of reducing side effects is to restrict the access of the drug, so that it is only administered to the site of required action. In the case of the treatment of asthma for example, the administration of steroids as aerosols rather than an as oral medication has led to a considerable reduction in side effects (Hopkins, 1999).

A third possibility is the use of drug targeting, an area in which considerable research is being carried out by pharmaceutical companies. An example of this approach is the use of salbutamol, rather than isoprenaline, to treat asthma. Both drugs have the required effect on the small air passages in the lungs, i.e. relaxation, but isoprenaline is not as selective as salbutamol (it is an agonist at both $\beta_1$ and $\beta_2$ adrenoceptors, whilst salbutamol is active mainly at $\beta_2$ adrenoceptors), and so produces side effects in the form of an increased heart rate. By using drugs that are selective for one receptor subtype, side effects can be minimised, although not cut out entirely as selectivity for a particular subtype is never 100%.

## Polypharmacy

A method used by many practitioners to deal with a side effect is to prescribe another drug to counteract it. This is often the case with, for example, morphine, where a laxative is prescribed to treat the constipation it causes. This can lead to a 'prescribing cascade', in which a drug is prescribed that causes a side effect, another drug is prescribed to combat the side effect, and the second drug causes further side effects (Reid & Crome, 1997). Constipation, nausea, confusion, headaches, and dizziness are all symptoms that are frequently the result of medication rather than new disease. The danger of this approach is that the patient ends up on multiple drugs, which is termed polypharmacy. This term does not simply mean that a patient is taking numerous drugs; instead, it implies that more drugs are being given than is clinically justified. Indicators of polypharmacy include using:

i.   a drug to treat an adverse effect
ii.  duplicate medications in the same drug category
iii. drugs contraindicated for use with the client group
iv.  medications that have no apparent indication
v.   inappropriate dosages
vi.  interacting medications concurrently (French, 1996).

Polypharmacy is common in the elderly and this might partly explain why research has found that those over 65 years of age experience more preventable adverse drug events than younger people (Thomas & Brennan, 2000).

Although many adverse drug reactions are predictable, as Table 5.1 indicates some are not at present, especially the bizarre ones, which are due to characteristics of the patient rather than the drug. For example, many drugs undergo acetylation in the liver as part of their metabolism. The enzyme that controls this reaction, N-acetyltransferase, occurs in several forms (i.e. it is polymorphic). Depending on how active the enzyme is, individuals can be either slow or fast acetylators. Slow acetylators do not remove certain drugs very quickly from their system, so if given normal doses of a drug, its concentration can build up in the tissues and cause toxicity. Thus, for example, if a slow acetylator receives procainamide, which is commonly used after a heart attack, the patient has a 60% chance of developing a liver disease which could be fatal (Schmidt, 1998). It is hoped that in the future, as our knowledge of the human genome increases, we will be able to carry out DNA tests on a patient and then tailor the drugs to the individual patient's genotype.

## Alternative and complementary therapies

As public concern with mainstream medicine has grown, many people have turned to the use of alternative and complementary therapies, including herbal medications. These plant-based remedies often consist of mixtures of diverse herbal ingredients of varying potency. The potency depends on the part of the plant used, e.g. root, stem, leaves and fruits, the time of the year it is picked, and the actual species of plant used, e.g. Ginseng may refer to many *Panax* and *Eleutherococcus* species (D'Arcy, 1993). These remedies are not generally used in orthodox western medicine because they do not fit with the reductionist paradigm of the conventional practitioner, who prefers drugs with only one or two active ingredients of known potency.

It is estimated that 30 to 45% of Americans now use herbal products as medications (Cohen, 1998; Lee & Horne, 2001), and spending on herbal products in the United Kingdom is now over £40 million a year (Vickers & Zollman, 1999). When McLesky and colleagues asked 979 patients about to undergo surgery about their use of herbal remedies and nutraceuticals (supplements not derived from plants) 170 (17.4%) of the patients reported taking such products (Larkin, 1999). The most frequently used herbs were ginkgo (*Ginkgo biloba*) (32.4%), ginseng (*Panax* and *Eleutherococcus* species) (26.5%), and garlic (*Allium sativum*) (26.5%), whilst the most commonly used nutraceuticals included glucosamine (17%), chromium picolinate (17%) and chondrition (12%).

Part of the reason for the move to herbal remedies is that the people (including medical practitioners) believe that because these preparations are 'natural' and have a long history of use, they are also free of risk (D'Arcy 1993; Cohen *et al.*, 2000). This is reinforced when they are so easily available in supermarkets, health food shops, and chemists. However, herbal remedies have much in common with modern drugs, many of which are also derived from plants, and both have proven therapeutic effects (see Barrett *et al.* (1999) for a review of the evidence supporting the benefits of herbal medicines). Nevertheless, just as modern drugs can be iatrogenic, so can herbal medicines, and they probably present a greater risk of adverse effects than any other complementary therapy (Vickers & Zollman, 1999). There are numerous case reports of serious adverse effects from herbal remedies, and in most cases these were self-prescribed and bought over the counter rather than prescribed by a registered practitioner. Table 5.2 gives examples of potentially serious adverse effects that can occur with use of herbal remedies.

Modern drugs have generally undergone extensive testing for therapeutic and adverse effects in a formalised manner. However, it must be noted that the extensiveness of this testing must be questioned when an estimated 80% of prescription drugs have not been tested, and hence are not licensed for use, in children (Cote *et al.*, 1996). Herbal remedies, which are not regulated in the same manner as orthodox drugs, are not required to undergo systematic testing, and so our knowledge of their potential adverse effects and interactions is limited. Within Britain and the United States, they are considered as dietary supplements rather than as drugs. Consequently, companies selling them cannot make any claims about their therapeutic effects, and they give no advice about their adverse effects.

As has already been indicated, herbal remedies are not standardised, and their effects are often the result of multiple active ingredients. For example St John's Wort (*Hypericum perforatum*) contains at least 10 constituents or groups of components that may contribute to its pharmacological effects, including naphthodianthroms, flavenoids, xanthose and bioflavonoids (Miller, 1998). Consequently, there is wide inter-product and intra-product (lot-to-lot) variation in the composition of active constituents.

Herbal medicines are not required to undergo the same quality checks as conventional drugs for purity or potency and so they may

**Table 5.2** Examples of serious adverse effects of herbal remedies.

| Herb | Potential adverse effects |
|---|---|
| Ginkgo (*Ginkgo biloba*) | Subarachnoid haemorrhage and subdural haematoma (Gilbert, 1997; Vale, 1998) |
| Ma huang (*Ephedra* species) | Seizures, arrhythmia's, myocardial infarction, stroke, death (Cupp, 1999) |
| Ginseng (This vernacular term refers to many *Panax* and *Eleutherococcus* species) | Vaginal bleeding and mastalgia (Punnonen & Lukola, 1980; Greenspan, 1983) |
| Kava-kava (*Piper methysticum*) | Extrapyramidal effects (Schelosky *et al.*, 1995) |
| Nutmeg (*Myristicia fragans*) | Hallucinations, psychosis (Brown, 2000) |
| Yohimbine (*Pausinystalia yohimbe*) | Hypertension (Lacombiez *et al.*, 1989) |

be contaminated, adulterated or misidentified. For example, many Asian and Indian herbal remedies have been found to contain heavy metals such as lead, arsenic and mercury (Capriotti, 1999). One of the worst examples of contamination causing adverse effects occurred in the United States in 1989 where there was an outbreak of eosinophilia-myalgia syndrome (EMS) associated with the use of L-tryptophan, an over-the-counter dietary supplement used for weight loss (Anon, 1999). Over 1500 cases of EMS, including 38 deaths, were reported. More than 95% of the cases were traced to an individual Japanese supplier. Researchers found some trace-level impurities, suggesting that a contaminated batch of L-tryptophan contributed to the outbreak.

## Interactions between conventional drugs and herbal remedies

As most consumers believe herbal medicines are harmless, they have no qualms in taking them in conjunction with prescribed conventional medicines. In addition, many immigrants in the UK have their own traditional medicinal practices, which they commonly combine with orthodox medical care (D'Arcy, 1993; Lomax *et al.*, 2001). Both these practices can lead to iatrogenic harm through herb–drug interactions. The problem of interactions between herbal remedies and mainstream drugs is increased because 30% of patients do not inform their doctor that they are using them (Eisenberg *et al.*, 1993). This is because patients either do not consider herbal remedies as 'drugs', and so when asked for a history of their medications they do not mention them, or alternatively they are reticent about mentioning them for fear of a negative response from the health care worker (Lomax *et al.*, 2001). Table 5.3 gives some examples of important potential interactions between herbal preparations and conventional drugs. In order to minimise potential interactions, it is vital that clinicians include questions about herbal remedies in their routine drug histories, and be informed rather than judgemental about their use.

Support for such an argument can be found in relation to the herbal antidepressant, St John's Wort. There are few doubts about the efficacy of it as a herbal antidepressant but possible interactions with conventional drugs are a growing concern (Ernst, 1999), although it causes fewer adverse effects than synthetic antidepressants (Linde *et al.*, 1996). The complexity facing those in health care who increasingly have to balance orthodox drug therapy with the herbal remedies that people are taking, is that both groups can and will interact. Not only is there the potential for them to interact within the drug/herbal remedy group, but also across the groups as described in Table 5.3. The task of those in health care increasingly appears to be to assist people using such therapies to balance the risks and maximise the benefits. That means understanding the possible interactions between conventional drug and herbal therapies.

## Compliance and concordance

### Compliance

Long-term medication compliance is around the 50% mark (Haynes *et al.*, 1979), and even where there are grave consequences of non-compliance as in the case of glaucoma and blindness, renal transplant and organ rejection, and the patient understands this, significant non-compliance has been reported in as many as 20% of patients (Laurence *et al.*, 1997). Patient non-compliance can involve underuse and overuse of medication and may be deliberate or unintentional. Table 5.4 identifies the five most common forms of patient medication non-compliance and possible iatrogenic harm that can result.

Overcoming non-compliance in relation to drug therapy is

**Table 5.3** Examples of important potential interactions between herbal preparations and conventional drugs (Miller, 1998; Larkin, 1999; Fugh-Berman 2000).

| Herb | Conventional drug | Potential adverse effect |
|---|---|---|
| Purple cone flower/ Echinacea (*E. purpurea, E. pallida, E. angustifolia*) (used for 8 weeks +) | Amiodarone, anabolic steroids, ketoconazole, methotrexate | Hepatotoxicity |
| Ma huang (*Ephedra* species) | Antidepressants, antihypertensives | Tachycardia, hypertension |
| Ginseng (This vernacular term refers to many *Panax* and *Eleutherococcus* species) | Warfarin | Bleeding |
| Ginseng (This vernacular term refers to many *Panax* and *Eleutherococcus* species) | Digoxin | Bradycardia |
| Kava-kava (*Piper methysticum*) | Benzodiazepines | Excessive sedation, coma |
| Karela or bitter melon (*Momordica charantia*) | Biguanides, insulin, sulphonylureas | Hypoglycaemia |
| Liquorice (*Glycyrrhiza glabra*) | Spironolactone | Reduced diuretic effect |
| St John's Wort (*Hypericum perforatum*) | Serotonin-reuptake inhibitors | Serotonin syndrome |
| St John's Wort (*Hypericum perforatum*) | Anaesthetics, narcotics | Excessive sedation |
| Valerian (*Valeriana officinalis*) | Barbiturates | Excessive sedation |

difficult. The health care worker is left with the dilemma of respecting patients' autonomy and right not to follow prescribed treatments while ensuring that limited health resources are not wasted on clients who put themselves at risk of increased morbidity

**Table 5.4**   Iatrogenic harm that can result from non-compliance.

| Top 5 forms of drug non-compliance (Hughes, 1998) | Examples of possible iatrogenic harm caused by non-compliance |
|---|---|
| Not having the prescription filled | Not obtaining immuno-suppressive drugs resulting in organ rejection |
| Taking the incorrect dose | Paracetamol overdose leading to liver failure |
| Taking the medicine at the wrong times | Taking diuretics in the evening, leading to urinary incontinence |
| Forgetting to take the medicine | Pregnancy due to omission of oral contraceptive |
| Stopping the medicine too soon | Antibiotic-resistant infection due to incomplete course of antibiotics; Addison's crisis due to stopping steroids. |

through non-compliance. The work of Wright and Morgan (1990) illustrates the complexities of compliance in exploring the reactions of a number of young people with cystic fibrosis to prescribed drug regimes. The people in the study were seen to use their behaviour in relation to adherence to prescribed drug regimes, to exert power in the patient–doctor relationship. Furthermore, their shortened life expectancy led some to use prescribed drugs in ways that gained them short-term body image benefits but in doses that caused concern to the medical and nursing staff – doses that would generally be considered extreme. Such strategies frequently led to these people being labelled as 'problem patients'. Doctors and nurses need to discover what patients are really doing with their medication and use this information to advise patients against any dangerous practices and in negotiation with the patient devise more acceptable, but effective and therapeutic regimens. This, the Audit Commission (2001) believes, can be aided by promoting the use of patient self-administration of medicines within hospital settings.

Non-compliance is not only a patient issue, as some patients who are dependent on nurses to administer their medications frequently fail to receive drugs as prescribed. This may take the form of overusage of drugs, e.g. excessive use of analgesics and tranquil-lisers in intensive care leading to drug dependency (Taylor, 1999) and inappropriate use of antibiotics and antiseptics leading to antibiotic resistance (DoH, 1999a; Clark 2000). In fact, Scott (1997) argues that antibiotic prescribing is the single most abused privilege of doctors, for the problem of resistance is an example of drug-related iatrogenic harm on a grand scale. It has led to infections like methicillin-resistant *Staphylococcus aureus* (MRSA) becoming rife in our hospitals, causing increased morbidity and mortality in patients and absorbing huge sums of the NHS budget in preventive and treatment measures. The British Medical Association (1997) has urged government to fund educational campaigns aimed at both clinicians and the public in order to promote effective drug usage.

## Concordance

More recently, concordance has superseded the concept of patient compliance (Marinker, 1997). This change represents an acknowledgement of the importance of understanding the patient's/client's perspective on their medication and its perceived impact on their health. Individuals will frequently adjust their medication as their health improves or deteriorates. A good example of such adjustments can be found in self-medication for asthma. The study by Lomax *et al.* (2001) which involved in-depth interviews with 107 people from a range of ethnic groups, found that 'leaving off' medication, reducing or stopping asthma drugs when their asthma improved, was common. Lomax *et al.* argued that to understand reasons for the lack of adherence to prescribed drug regimes it is necessary to go beyond the traditional division of patients into compliers and non-compliers. Furthermore, a relationship of partnership between those in health care and the patient or client, as opposed to one of the instructive professional expecting compliance, is preferred by those on medication and they are, within such a relationship, more likely to disclose any complementary medications they are using.

## *Drug errors*

Non-compliance with policies and procedures by staff can result in drug errors (Fuqua and Stevens, 1988). These can be defined as preventable prescribing, dispensing or administration mistakes (Cousins & Upton, 1993), and they are frighteningly common events. In the community, drug errors account for 25% of litigation claims against general practitioners (DoH, 2000a). In UK hospitals around 1 in 20 drug doses is given incorrectly or omitted (Table 5.5), and in one week in the North Thames Region, pharmacists intercepted over 900 prescribing errors that they thought could have

**Table 5.5**  Observation-based studies of medication administration errors in UK hospitals (from Kelly, J. (2000) *Adverse Drug Effects: A nursing concern.* Whurr Publishers Ltd, London. With permission of the publishers).

| Study | Doses observed | Error rate |
|---|---|---|
| Dean *et al.*, 1995 | 2756 | 3.0% |
| Ridge *et al.*, 1995 | 3312 | 3.5% |
| Gethins, 1996 | 2000 | 3.2% |
| Cavell and Hughes, 1997 | 1206 | 5.7% |
| Ho *et al.*, 1997 | 2170 | 5.5% |
| Ogden *et al.*, 1997 | 2973 | 5.5% |
| Taxis *et al.*, 1998 | 842 | 8.0% |

resulted in severe morbidity or death (Barber & Dean, 1998). However, as few outcome studies have been carried out in the UK it is hard to know how much harm would actually have occurred. Outcome studies are common in the USA. An examination of all US death certificates between 1983 and 1993 identified that there had been a 2.57-fold increase in deaths from medication errors (from 2876 in 1983 to 7391 in 1993), with 1195 of the deaths in 1993 being inpatient deaths (Phillips *et al.*, 1998).

A review of coroner's records in Birmingham concluded that about a fifth of deaths relating to prescribing and administering drugs were due to errors, and that these deaths are more easily prevented than those due to adverse drug reactions (Ferner & Whittington, 1994). Table 5.6 gives examples of the causes of common medication errors as identified in the literature. In order to prevent these errors and develop safer systems it is necessary to establish the risks of the current system, but it is not known how many medication errors really occur within most hospitals in the UK as there is considerable under-detection and under-reporting (Cousins & Upton, 1993). This is particularly the case in nursing where the response by management to nurses' admitting drug errors is often punitive (Arndt, 1994; Bassett, 1998). The NMC (2002) has been critical of this approach and has called for a more open and sensitive culture, for if we cannot learn from our errors, the same mistake will be made repeatedly and patients will suffer. To prevent this happening requires reporting of not just errors that have occurred, but also near misses. A tragic example of our failure to learn from our mistakes is provided by the fact that more than 14 patients have died or been paralysed since 1985 because a drug has been wrongly administered by spinal injection (DoH, 2000a).

**Table 5.6** Common causes of medication errors (adapted from Kelly, J. (2000) *Adverse Drug Effects: A nursing concern*. Whurr Publishers Ltd, London. With permission of the publishers).

| | |
|---|---|
| i. | Corporate/look-alike packaging produced by drug companies (Knowles, 1998) |
| ii. | Similar drug names, e.g. carbimazole/carbamazepine (Boyce, 1998) |
| iii. | Use of abbreviations, e.g. AZT for both zidovudine and azathioprine (Ambrosini *et al.*, 1992) |
| iv. | Illegible handwriting (Lyons *et al.*, 1998) |
| v. | Duplicate prescribing, e.g. drug prescribed both as a 'regular' and 'as required' (Gethins, 1996) |
| vi. | Trailing zeros, e.g. writing 1.0 mg rather than 1 mg (Davis, 1994a) |
| vii. | Inaccurate dosage calculations (Gladstone, 1995) |
| viii. | Inadequately trained personnel (lack of knowledge about the drug and/or patient) (Leape *et al.*, 1995) |
| ix. | Single-handed drug administration (Cohen *et al.*, 1994) |
| x. | Lapses in individual performance often due to interruptions during drug rounds (Davis, 1994b) |
| xi. | Work load, understaffing, poor skill mix (ASHP, 1993; Schulmeister, 1999) |
| xii. | Shift patterns (O'Shea, 1999) |
| xiii. | Verbal orders (Fuqua & Stevens, 1988) |

The National Health Service must recognise that human error is inevitable no matter how knowledgeable and careful health care workers are (see Chapter 2). Research specifically focused on health care systems suggests that as many as 70% of adverse incidents are preventable (DoH, 2000a). However, although errors can be minimised they will never completely be eliminated – particularly where high volumes of activity occur. For example, it has been estimated that a 600 bed teaching hospital with a 99.9% error free drug ordering, dispensing and administration rate will experience 4000 drug errors a year (Leape, 1994). If human error cannot be prevented, then the NHS must move away from a person-centred approach, which pivots on disciplinary measures, to a systems approach, which sees human error as a consequence, not a cause of the failure. This approach uses a technique developed in the aerospace industry and known as 'failure mode and effects analysis', which identifies potential mistakes and determines whether the consequences of those mistakes would be tolerable or intolerable (see also Chapter 2). Where potential effects are unacceptable actions are taken to eliminate the possibility of error, trap any error

**Table 5.7** Systems based solutions of medication errors (adapted from Kelly, J. (2000) *Adverse Drug Effects: A nursing concern.* Whurr Publishers Ltd, London. With permission of the publishers).

| | |
|---|---|
| i. | Legally require drug companies to avoid similar sounding names for their products and to review their packaging (ASHP, 1993) |
| ii. | Intelligent computer system for drug prescribing (Cavell & Hughes, 1997; Bates, 2000) |
| iii. | Participation of pharmacists in ward rounds (Leape *et al.*, 1999) |
| iv. | Computerised drug distribution systems (Davis, 1994c) |
| v. | No interruptions of staff giving out medications (Cooper, 1995) |
| vi. | Not accepting verbal orders for drugs (UKCC, 2000) |
| vii. | Clear guidelines for defining what constitutes a drug error and what specific action should be taken in the event (Cousins & Upton, 1993) |
| viii. | Development of documentation which collects relevant and detailed information regarding the circumstances and effect of each drug error together with a database of all drug incidents to enable continuous monitoring and the early identification of trends and variations (Cousins & Upton, 1993) |

before it reaches a patient or minimise the consequences of the error when potential errors cannot be eliminated.

This approach could be applied to drug management in order to prevent errors and accidents (Cohen *et al.*, 1994). For example, potassium chloride for injection in vials of 1.5 g (20 mmol of potassium) per 10 ml, has been involved in more fatal medication errors than any other drug (Davis, 1995). Failure mode and effects analysis identifies the answer to this problem as removal of the possibility of error. This is achieved by removing potassium chloride for injection concentrate from ward environments and stocking minibags of potassium chloride injection instead. Other examples of systems-based solutions to drug errors are given in Table 5.7.

## The role of the drug companies

It will be noted that in the main it is the health service that needs to instigate changes to reduce drug errors. However, the other major party is the drug companies. They produce drugs in corporate packaging so that packets have the same colours, fonts and general presentation, making it easy in an emergency to select a packet of the wrong drug. To add to the confusion drug companies often give their drugs names which are very similar to other very different drugs, e.g. phentermine and phentolamine. Similar sounding drug names are believed to cause one in four prescribing errors and the consequence can be disastrous: a patient given amrinone (a phosphodiesterase inhibitor) instead of amiodarone is likely to develop a worse arrhythmia and die (Boyce, 1998). At present, the European Agency for the Evaluation of Medicinal Products does warn companies that a drug name must have three or more 'distinguishing letters'. However, this is clearly not enough. Either the drug companies should act responsibly and make their products safer, or changes to the law must be made to force them to be safer. Practitioners can also take their own measures. One such measure would be for hospital pharmacies to stock different doses of a drug from different drug companies so that the only packaging difference is not the drug dosage itself.

## *Nurse prescribing*

It is clear that drugs of all types are a major cause of iatrogenic harm, and further action is required to minimise this risk through safer prescribing, dispensing and administering. Until recently nurses were only involved with the last part of this process, but with the advent of nurse prescribing in the UK their role in the prevention of drug induced iatrogenic harm is going to increase. Recommendations for nurse prescribing were first made in the Cumberlege Report (DHSS, 1986) when it was suggested that community nurses should be able to prescribe 'prescription-only medicines' from a limited list. This was reinforced by the Crown Report (DoH, 1989) which recommended that 'suitably qualified nurses working in the community should be able – in clearly defined circumstances – to prescribe from a limited list of items and to adjust timing, and dosage of medicine within a set protocol'. In 1992 the Medicinal Products: Prescribing by Nurses Act was passed enabling nurses in the community to prescribe by identifying them as 'appropriate practitioners'. The Pharmaceutical Services Regulations were later passed in 1994 together with the Medicines Order, the former to allow pharmacists in the community to dispense medicines prescribed by nurses, and the latter to set the limitations of the prescribing powers of nurses. Thus, community nurses can prescribe a limited range of drugs from the *Nurse Prescribers' Formulary* provided the nurse:

i.   is a first-level registered nurse with a district nurse, midwifery or health visitor qualification
ii.  works within a primary care setting

iii. has successfully completed a nurse prescribing programme
iv. is registered with the NMC as a nurse prescriber
v. is authorised/required by their employer to prescribe.

Full implementation of nurse prescribing was to be implemented by April 1998 (DoH, 1996) and every Trust and Health Authority in England commissioned training programmes, changing nurses' job descriptions and negotiating protocols. By March 2001, it was esti- mated 26,000 district nurses and health visitors would have pre- scribing authority (Gooch, 1999).

The publication of the second Crown report (DoH, 1999b) added impetus to the drive for nurse prescribing by concluding that doc- tors are not the only health professionals who take legitimate responsibility for making clinical assessments leading to a diag- nosis. Crown recommended a two-tier approach with independent prescribers who would diagnose and prescribe, and dependent prescribers who would meet the needs of patients with a known diagnosis. This was followed in October 2000 by the government's announcement of radical plans to extend nurse prescribing (DoH, 2000b) with five options being offered for discussion (see Table 5.8). This move supported the NHS Plan (DoH, 2000c) which specified that most nurses should be qualified (under patient group direc- tions) to prescribe or supply medicines by 2004 (DoH, 2000d).

Frances Pickersgill, RCN policy adviser, was quoted as saying 'it would be far-reaching to go for option five, but we should go for the best that is on offer and cope with the risk management and accountability later' (Parish, 2000 p. 5). This was perhaps a little like 'putting the cart before the horse', and is not a safe approach in the light of the evidence presented here, nor does it give nurses credi- bility with their medical colleagues. There is a deep unease amongst doctors who believe that if nurses are going to have full access to all the drugs in the *British National Formulary* this would require equal training to that received by a doctor, or it would make doctors' training a nonsense (Jeffery, 2001). The problems about knowledge levels are returned to later in this chapter.

The second issue that Pickersgill's statement raises is, 'best' for whom? Nurse prescribing can only be supported if it is going to benefit patients and allow nurses to be more effective at enhancing health. It should not be another step towards taking nursing towards a medical model and diverting attention from the core element of nursing, which is caring for the patients. There seems to be considerable pressure for nurses to take on roles from doctors, and leave the traditional hands-on care to health care assistants

**Table 5.8** The five options for extending the nursing formulary (Department of Health, 2000b).

| | |
|---|---|
| **Option 1** | No change. Suitably trained nurses continue with current formulary, with additional medicines being added when approved by the Nurse Prescribers' Formulary sub-committee. |
| **Option 2** | Expand the formulary to include all over-the-counter (General Sales List (GSL)) and Pharmacy (P) (medicines available from a pharmacist without a prescription) medicines. |
| **Option 3** | Expand the formulary to include GSL and P medicines, as well as some prescription-only medicines (POM) to treat conditions such as asthma and diabetes. Nurse prescribers would have to demonstrate competency to prescribe items. |
| **Option 4** | Expand the formulary to include GSL, P and POM medicines, except controlled drugs. Again, nurse prescribers would have to demonstrate competency to prescribe items. |
| **Option 5** | Expand the formulary to include GSL, P and POM medicines. Other drugs could be prescribed by suitably trained nurses, including some controlled drugs, once legislative changes had been made. Each nurse would have to demonstrate competency to prescribe items. |

(Castledine, 2001). Nurse prescribing significantly blurs the boundaries between nurses and doctors. However, most nurses maintain that they do not want to be doctors, and see themselves instead as 'providing informed holistic care which enables a patient to manage their illness once a diagnosis has been made, whereas doctors see their role as being about diagnosis, management, investigation and long term medical care' (Jeffery, 2001 p. 4).

In support of nurse prescribing is the fact that many nurses are already involved in this process, although they do not actually write out prescriptions, and thus nurse prescribing is merely legitimising existing practices. For example, in many hospitals a nurse will assess a wound, identify the best dressing and then get it from the store cupboard. In the community, if a nurse requires a similar dressing for a patient she has to ask a doctor to prescribe it for her. Furthermore, in the community, nurses will frequently see patients and identify that the patient has a medical problem that needs drug treatment, for example a wound infection, and the GP will rely on the nurse's judgement, prescribing an antibiotic without seeing the patient. Similarly, in hospital many nurses advise junior and senior medical staff on what and how much to prescribe for patients (Castledine, 2000).

Another anomaly that nurse prescribing will abate is that patients can walk into their local supermarket and buy over-the-counter medications such as cimetidine. Yet, if a nurse identifies that a patient requires this drug she either has to ask a doctor to write a prescription for it, or encourage the patient to buy the drug. Furthermore, with the development of nurse consultants and specialist nurses, particularly those working in walk-in clinics and accident and emergency units, the need for nurse prescribing has become more clear.

Recognising the need to extend nurse prescribing in order to help break down professional barriers, increase access to services, and improve patient care, but at the same time exercising prudence, the Department of Health judiciously decided on Option 3 (DoH, 2002a, see Table 5.8). The intention is also to expand nurse prescribing across all sectors, including both primary and secondary care, as well as nurse-led services. The decision on which nurses should receive training will be taken locally based on service need, which of course might include a shortage of medical staff, and benefit to patients. In preparation for the new role there will be a three-month degree level programme comprising 25 taught days, some self-directed learning, a period of supervised practice under the guidance of a medical practitioner, and assessment of practical and theoretical competencies (DoH, 2002b).

This is very modest compared with the USA where most states require nurses to have a Masters degree in their speciality, complete 500 hours of supervised clinical practice, and sit a four hour examination for certification by the American Nurses' Association (Duffin, 2001). The new nurse prescribing courses began early in 2002 (at 30 April 2002 over 500 nurses had completed, or were taking, the preparation courses) and it is anticipated that 10,000 new nurses will be trained by 2004 (Mullally, 2001). This timescale has put pressure on teaching establishments to prepare good quality courses which will turn out safe practitioners. Current prescribers and those who qualify in future through the health visitor or district nurse specialist practitioner programmes will continue to prescribe from the original *Nurse Prescriber's Formulary*, unless they undertake the new training. Thus, there will be a confusing two level system of independent prescribers, as well as the planned dependent or supplementary prescribers (who are able to prescribe after an independent prescriber has assessed a patient and drawn up a treatment plan (DoH, 2002c)).

## Drug calculations

If it is accepted that nurse prescribing can improve patient care, and certainly it would appear that some patients think it does (Brooks *et al.*, 2001), then the question is not so much whether nurses should prescribe, as whether they are able to do so. There is concern that some nurses lack numeracy and cognitive skills and so are not fully competent to administer medications, let alone prescribe them. It was recognised by the UKCC, mainly through misconduct trials that patients' lives were being put at risk because some nurses are very poor at mathematics and give widely inaccurate measures of drugs (Duffin, 2000).

According to Bryn Davis, a UKCC member and former dean of a school of nursing in Wales, the GCSE maths exam – a compulsory entry requirement for training – is failing to prepare nurses for complex drug calculations (Coombes, 2000). The use of calculators does not necessarily solve the problem, as for many nurses the main area of difficulty is 'setting up' the problem in order to do the arithmetic (Gillham & Chu, 1995; Cartwright, 1996). Neither does the use of a calculator question whether the answer is sensible, and many nurses are unable to recognise if the calculated dose is out by a factor of 10. Some nurses, particularly senior ones, think that it is a sign of professional competence if their work is not checked, and hospitals support this approach by advocating a single-handed drug administration policy, sometimes even in high risk areas such as paediatrics. These matters ought to be revisited, utilising the evidence and guidance available from the literature on error and error reduction.

Part of the solution to this problem is to follow the road taken by some universities that include numeracy skills teaching within their curriculum and insist on a 100% score in mathematical competency before nurses are allowed to qualify (Truman, 2000). It might be argued that insisting on zero tolerance at student level will lead to potentially excellent nurses failing to qualify, but this is perhaps preferable to allowing potentially fatal mistakes to be made. The need to recruit more nurses may also prevent the use of such strict criteria.

A recent editorial in the *Nursing Times* suggested that we should not get 'hot under the collar' about nurses' inability to do sums, as most high-profile drug errors have not been caused by nurses but by doctors, anaesthetists and pharmacists (Anon, 2000). This comment begs the question whether this state of affairs will change with nurse prescribing. However, it also has to be asked whether the research into nurses' mathematical ability is valid. How are students being tested on their ability to do drug calculations? Poor performance in a written mathematics test does not necessarily predict a lack of later competence in nursing mathematics required in the workplace where there are visual cues such as the drug and the syringe to aid the nurse in her calculations (Cartwright, 1996; Hutton, 1998). Similarly, passing a theoretical test, even one of some complexity, does not necessarily mean that the student will be accurate when performing in the practice setting.

## Do nurses have the necessary knowledge?

As well as issues with mathematical ability, there is concern that '…as nursing has striven to acquire professional autonomy, the biological sciences have been marginalised in the teaching and practice of nursing' (Jordan & Potter, 1999 p. 46). If this is the case then nurses are going to have difficulty administering drugs, let alone prescribing them, for the NMC (2002, p. 6) states that when *administering* a drug the nurse, '…must know the therapeutic uses of the medicine to be administered, its normal dosage, side-effects, precautions and contra-indications'. Theoretically this knowledge can be learnt by rote for all drugs that the nurse comes into contact with, or it can be gained by an understanding of how the body interacts with a drug (pharmacokinetics) and how the drug interacts with the body (pharmacodynamics). If nurses do not have a good grounding in biosciences they will be unable to understand pharmacology, and drug errors and other forms of unnecessary harm will be more likely to occur. A study by Leape *et al.* (1995) identified that the most common reason for drug errors was lack of knowledge, accounting for 29% of the 334 errors that occurred in a six-month period. Specifically in the administration of medications by nurses, lack of knowledge accounted for 15% of the problems.

The difficulties nurses have with biosciences lie in several areas. Students coming into nursing in the UK seem to have a poor grounding in human biology, and can find the biosciences taught during the first year of the pre-registration nursing course very difficult. The problem is compounded by the fact that the UKCC (1986) recommended that this part of the course focused on health rather than illness. Consequently, tutors attempt to teach normal anatomy and physiology without mentioning disease. As a result, students do not necessarily see the relevance of what they are being taught as they cannot relate the theory to their clinical practice which, as described earlier in this book, tends to be biomedical and therefore disease focused. Furthermore, many nurse teachers admit to having a poor knowledge of biosciences, especially pharmacology (Courtenay, 1991), and few hold degrees in biological sciences, favouring instead degrees in behavioural subjects. Because tutors feel inadequately prepared to teach biological science they may use self-directed teaching and learning methods, which are perceived by students as being ineffective (Courtenay, 1991). The fact that nurse teachers can get to what is seen as eminent positions in nursing without knowledge of the biosciences also serves to convey the message to students that you can be a successful nurse without understanding biosciences.

## Conclusion

Orthodox drugs and herbal remedies both have therapeutic and adverse effects. The latter can lead to iatrogenic harm, and for many patients the fear of this potential harm is one of the main reasons why they frequently choose not to take the medications that they are prescribed, leading to potentially poor control of their disease and increased morbidity and mortality. Failure to prescribe, dispense and administer drugs correctly can further increase the risk of injury. However, the reduction of iatrogenic harm is everyone's concern, and it can only be achieved if prescribers and patients alike recognise that drugs have the potential to do great harm as well as great good. Thus, they should not be used as a panacea for all our problems, but should be prescribed, dispensed and administered with knowledge and skill.

Due to the close relationship nurses have with their patients, they are well placed to detect adverse drug effects early and act to deal with them before harm comes to the patient. They are also well placed to negotiate and monitor compliance and concordance. However, in order for nurses to play this crucial role there needs to be more emphasis during pre- and post-registration nurse education on health, disease and pharmacology, on taking a history and making an assessment, and on medicines management. If nurses wish to extend their role safely and prescribe drugs as well as administer them, they must ensure that they are competent to do so, as their patients' welfare must be their prime concern. If they have any doubts about their competence, and many nurses have (Duffin

2001), they should not allow themselves to be pressurised into this new role. Furthermore, nurse managers and educators must guarantee that the push for nurse prescribing is for the benefit of the patient and not the organisation. They must also ensure that nurses get the quality education and support they require to fulfil this new task; for of all the changes to the role of the nurse, the expansion of nurse prescribing has the greatest potential for harm.

## Reducing harm with drug therapy

> In order to minimise unnecessary harm from drug therapy the nurse should:
>
> i.   consider whether the risks of withholding drug treatment are greater than the risks of the treatment itself
> ii.  ensure that the patient has been fully assessed, including all their prescribed drugs, over-the-counter medication and complementary therapies
> iii. ensure that both the health care worker and the patient fully understand how to use a medication correctly and the problems that may ensue if this does not occur
> iv.  strive for concordance and informed consent
> v.   ensure that drug errors and near misses are fully reported so that system can be put in place to minimise the chance of further errors occurring
> vi.  take responsibility for their own learning and ensure that they are competent to administer and prescribe drugs safely and legally
> vii. seek to question polypharmacy and poor prescription practices.

## *References*

Ambrosini, M. T., Mandler, H. D. & Wood, C. A. (1992) AZT: zidovudine or azathioprine? *The Lancet.* **339**, 935.

ASHP (American Society of Hospital Pharmacists) (1993) ASHP guidelines on preventing medication errors in hospitals. *American Journal of Hospital Pharmacy.* **50**, 305–314.

Anon. (1999) Are your chronically ill patients turning to herbs? *Disease State Management.* **5**, 66–70.

Anon. (2000) Getting hot under the collar about how good nurses are at maths doesn't add up. *Nursing Times.* **96**, (24) 3.

Arndt, M. (1994) Nurses' medication errors. *Journal of Advanced Nursing.* **19**, 519–526.

Audit Commission (2001) *A Spoonful of Sugar: Medicines management in NHS hospitals.* Audit Commission, London.

Barber, N. & Dean, B. (1998) The incidence of medication errors and ways to reduce them. *Clinical Risk.* **4**, 103–106.

Barrett, B., Keifer, D. & Rabago, D. (1999) Assessing the risks and benefits of herbal medicine: an overview of scientific evidence. *Alternative Therapies.* **5**, 40–49.

Bassett, S. (1998) The carrot beats the stick. *Nursing Management.* **5**, 6–7.

Bates, D. W. (2000) Using information technology to reduce rates of medication errors in hospitals. *British Medical Journal.* **32**, 788–791.

Boyce, N. (1998) It sounds like a prescription chaos. *New Scientist.* **160**, 28.

British Medical Association (1997) 'BMA warns that rising drug resistance is a major public health threat'. News release. *Lords Select Committee Enquiry into Antimicrobial Resistance.* BMA, London.

Brooks, N., Otway, C., Rashid, V., Kilty, L. & Maggs, C. (2001) Nurse prescribing: what do patients think? *Nursing Standard.* **15** (17), 33–38.

Brown, K. (2000) Scary spice. *New Scientist.* **168**, 53.

Capriotti, T. (1999) Exploring the 'herbal jungle'. *MEDSURG Nursing.* **8**, 53–63.

Cartwright, M. (1996) Numeracy needs of the beginning Registered Nurse. *Nurse Education Today.* **16**, 137–143.

Castledine, G. (2000) Nurse prescribing: the sensible way forward? *British Journal of Nursing.* **9**, 454.

Castledine, G. (2001) Millennial nursing: a look back on the past year. *British Journal of Nursing.* **10**, 63.

Cavell, G. F. & Hughes, D. K. (1997) Does computerised prescribing improve the accuracy of drug administration? *Pharmaceutical Journal.* **259**, 782–784.

Clark, L. (2000) Antibiotic resistance: a growing multifaceted problem. *British Journal of Nursing.* **9**, 225–230.

Cohen, M. R. (1998) Medication errors. *Nursing.* **28**, (11) 14.

Cohen, M. R., Senders, J. & Davis, N. M. (1994) Failure mode and effects analysis: a novel approach to avoiding dangerous medication errors and accidents. *Hospital Pharmacy.* **29**, 319–30.

Cohen, S. M., Rousseau, M. E. & Robinson, E. H. (2000) Therapeutic use of selected herbs. *Holistic Nursing Practice.* **14**, (3) 59–68.

Coombes, R. (2000) Nurses need a dose of maths. *Nursing Times.* **96**, (24) 4.

Cooper, M. (1995) Can a zero defects philosophy be applied to drug errors? *Journal of Advanced Nursing.* **21**, 487–491.

Cote, C. J., Kauffman, R. E., Troendle, G. J. & Lambert, G. H. (1996) Is the 'therapeutic orphan' about to be adopted? *Pediatrics.* **98**, 118–123.

Courtenay, M. (1991) A study of the teaching and learning of the biological sciences in nurse education. *Journal of Advanced Nursing.* **16**, 1110–1116.

Cousins, D. H. & Upton, D. R. (1993) Do you report medication errors? *Hospital Pharmacy Practice.* **3**, 376–378.

Cupp, M. J. (1999) Herbal remedies: adverse effects and drug interactions. *American Family Physician.* **59**, 1239–1244.

D'Arcy, P. F. (1991) Adverse reactions and interactions with herbal medi-cines. Part 1 – Adverse reactions. *Adverse Drug Reactions and Toxicological Reviews*. **10**, 189–208.

D'Arcy, P. F. (1993) Adverse reactions and interactions with herbal medi-cines. Part 2 – Drug interactions. *Adverse Drug Reactions and Toxicological Reviews*. **12**, 147–162.

Davis, N. (1994a) Beware of trailing zeros. *American Journal of Nursing*. **94**, (6) 17.

Davis, N. (1994b) Concentrating on interruptions. *American Journal of Nursing*. **94**, (3) 14.

Davis, N. (1994c) Can computers stop errors? *American Journal of Nursing*. **94**, (1) 14.

Davis, N. (1995) Potassium perils. *American Journal of Nursing*. **95**, (3) 14.

Dean, B. S., Allan, E. L., Barber, N. D. & Barker, K. N. (1995) Comparison of medication errors in an American and a British hospital. *American Journal of Health-System Pharmacy*. **52**, 2543–2549.

DoH (1989) *Report of the Advisory Group on Nursing Prescribing* (Crown Report). Department of Health, London.

DoH (1996) *Primary Care: Delivering the Future*. The Stationery Office, London.

DoH (1999a). *Resistance to antibiotics and other antimicrobial agents*. Health Service Circular. 1999/049. 5 March.

DoH (1999b) *Review of Prescribing, Supply and Administration of Medicines* (Crown Report II). Department of Health, London.

DoH (2000a) *An Organisation with a Memory. Report of an expert group on learning from adverse events in the NHS*. The Stationery Office, London.

DoH (2000b) *Consultation on Proposals to Extend Nurse Prescribing*. The Sta-tionery Office, London.

DoH (2000c) *The NHS Plan: A plan for investment, a plan for reform*. The Stationery Office, London.

DoH (2000d) *Patient Group Directions*. (England only HC2000/026). The Stationery Office, London.

DoH (2002a) *Items prescribable by nurses under the extended scheme*. www.doh.gov.uk/nurseprescribing/pomlisthtm

DoH (2002b) *Extending Independent Nurse Prescribing within the NHS in England*. The Stationery Office, London.

DoH (2002c) *Proposals for supplementary prescribing by nurses and pharmacists and proposed amendments to the Prescription Only Medicines (Human Use) Order 1997*. www.doh.gov.uk/supplementaryprescribing/faqs.htm

DHSS (1986) *Neighbourhood Nursing: A focus for care* (Cumberlege Report). Department of Health and Social Security, London.

Duffin, C. (2000) Poor standards of maths put patients' lives at risk. *Nursing Standard*. **14**, (39) 5.

Duffin, C. (2001) Slow and steady. *Nursing Standard*. **15**, 12–13.

Eisenberg, D. M., Kessler, R. C., Foster, C., Norlock, F. E. Calkins, D. R. & Delbanco, T. L. (1993) Unconventional medicine in the United States.

Prevalence, costs, and patterns of use. *New England Journal of Medicine.* **328**, 246–252.

Ernst, E. (1999) Second thought about safety of St John's Wort. *The Lancet.* **354**, 2014–2016.

Ferner, R. E. & Whittington, R. M. (1994) Coroner's cases of death due to errors of prescribing or giving medicines or to adverse drug reactions: Birmingham 1986–1991. *Journal of the Royal Society of Medicine.* **87**, 145–148.

French, D. G. (1996) Avoiding adverse drug reactions in the elderly patient: issues and strategies. *Nurse Practitioner.* **21**, (9) 90–105.

Fugh-Berman, A. (2000) Herb–drug interactions. *The Lancet.* **355**, 134–138.

Fuqua, R. A. & Stevens, K. R. (1988) What we know about medication errors: a literature review. *Journal of Nursing Quality Assurance.* **3**, 1–17.

Gethins, B. (1996) Wise up to medication errors. *Pharmacy in Practice.* **6**, 323–328.

Gilbert, G. J. (1997) Ginkgo biloba. *Neurology.* **48**, 1137.

Gillham, D. & Chu, S. (1995) An analysis of student nurses' medication calculation errors. *Contemporary Nurse.* **4** (2), 61–64.

Gladstone, J. (1995) Drug administration errors: a study into the factors underlying the occurrence and reporting of drug errors in a district general hospital. *Journal of Advanced Nursing.* **22**, 628–637.

Gooch, S. (1999) Nurse prescribing and the Crown review. *Professional Nurse.* **14**, 678–680.

Greenspan, E. (1983) Ginseng and vaginal bleeding. *Journal of the American Medical Association.* **249**, 2018.

Haynes, R. B., Taylor, D. W. & Sackett, D. L. (eds) (1979) *Compliance in Health Care.* Johns Hopkins University Press, Baltimore.

Ho, C. Y. W., Dean, B. S. & Barber, N. D. (1997) When do medication errors happen to hospital inpatients? *International Journal of Pharmacy Practice.* **5**, 91–96.

Hopkins, S. J. (1999) *Drugs and Pharmacology for Nurses.* Churchill Livingstone, London.

Hughes, S. (1998) Compliance with drug treatment in the elderly. *Prescriber.* **9**, 45–54.

Hutton, B. M. (1998) Nursing mathematics: the importance of application. *Nursing Standard.* **13** (11), 35–38.

Jeffery, C. (2001) Finding the right prescription. *RCN Magazine.* Spring, 3–5.

Jha, A. K., Kuperman, G. J., Teich, J. M., Leape, L., Shea, B., Rittenberg, E., Burdick, E., Seger, D. L., Vander Vleit, M. & Bates, D. W. (1998) Identifying adverse drug events: development of a computer-based monitor and comparison with chart review and stimulated voluntary report. *Journal of the American Medical Informatics Association.* **5**, 305–314.

Jordan, S. & Potter, N. (1999) Biosciences on the margin. *Nursing Standard.* **13**, (25) 46–48.

Kelly, J. (2000) *Adverse Drug Effects: A nursing concern.* Whurr, London.

Knowles, D. R. (1998) Supplying medicines safely. *Clinical Risk.* **4**, 107–109.

Lacombiez, L., Bensimon, G. & Isnad, F. (1989) Effect of yohimbine on blood pressure in patients with depression and orthostatic hypertension induced by clomipramine. *Clinical Pharmacology and Therapeutics.* **45**, 241–251.

Lambert, E. C. (1978) *Modern Medical Mistakes.* Indiana University Press, Bloomington.

Larkin, M. (1999) Surgery patients at risk from herb–anaesthesia interactions. *Lancet.* **354**, 1362.

Laurence, D. R., Bennett, P. N. & Brown M. J. (1997) *Clinical Pharmacology,* 8th edn. Churchill Livingstone, Edinburgh.

Lazarou, J., Pomeranz, B. H. & Corey, P. N. (1998) Incidence of adverse drug reactions in hospitalised patients. *Journal of the American Medical Association.* **279**, 1200–1205.

Leape, L. (1994) The preventability of medical injury. In: *Human Error in Medicine* (ed. M. S. Bogner), pp. 13–25. Lawrence Erlbaum Associates, Hove.

Leape, L. L., Bates, D. W., Cullen, D. J., Cooper, J., Demonaco, H. J., Gallivan, T., Hallisey, R., Ives, J., Laird, N. & Laffel, G. (1995) Systems analysis of adverse drug events. *Journal of the American Medical Association.* **274**, 35–43.

Leape, L., Cullen, D. J., Clapp, M. D., Burdick, E., Demonaco, H. J., Erickson, J. I. & Bates, D. W. (1999) Pharmacist participation on physician rounds and adverse drug events in the intensive care unit. *Journal of the American Medical Association.* **282**, 267–270.

Lee, S. J. & Horne, C. H. (2001) Herbal products and conventional medicines used by community-residing older women. *Journal of Advanced Nursing.* **33**, 51–59.

Linde, K., Ramirez, G., Mulrow, C. D., Pauls, A., Weidenhammer, W. & Melchart, D. (1996) St John's Wort for depression – an overview and meta-analysis of randomised clinical trials. *British Medical Journal.* **313**, 253–258.

Lomax, H., Brooks, F. & Mitchell, M. (2001) Understanding user health care strategies: experiences of asthma therapy among South Asians and White cultural groups. In: *New Beginnings: Towards Patient and Public Involvement in Primary Care?* (eds F. Brooks & S. Gillam), pp. 77–89. King's Fund, London.

Lyons, R., Payne, C., McCabe, M,. & Fielder, C. (1998) Legibility of doctors' handwriting: quantitative comparative study. *British Medical Journal.* **317**, 863–864.

Marinker, M. (1997) Personal paper: writing prescriptions is easy. *British Medical Journal.* **314**, 747.

Miller, L. G. (1998) Herbal medicinals: selected clinical considerations focusing on known potential drug–herb interactions. *Archives of International Medicine.* **158**, 2200–2211.

Mullally, S. (2001) Prescribing update. *Nursing Standard.* **15**, (45) 22.

Nursing & Midwifery Council (2002) *Guidelines for the administration of medicines.* NMC, London.

Ogden, D. A., Kinnear, M. & McArthur, D. M. (1997) A quantitative and qualitative evaluation of medication errors in hospital inpatients. *Pharmacy Practice Research.* Supplement to *Pharmaceutical Journal.* **259** (6968), R19.

O'Shea, E. (1999) Factors contributing to medication errors: a literature review. *Journal of Clinical Nursing.* **8**, 496–504.

Page, C. P., Curtis, M. J., Sutter, M. C., Walker, M. J. A. & Hoffman, B. B. (1997) *Integrated Pharmacology.* C.V. Mosby, London.

Parish, C. (2000) Government offers five options for prescribing. *Nursing Standard.* **15** (7), 5.

Phillips, D. P., Christenfeld, N. & Glynn, L. M. (1998) Increase in US medication-error deaths between 1983 and 1993. *The Lancet.* **351**, 643–644.

Punnonen, R. & Lukola, A. (1980) Oestrogen-like effects of ginseng. *British Medical Journal.* **281**, 1110.

Reid, J. & Crome, P. (1997) Polypharmacy: causes and effects in elderly patients. *Prescriber.* **8** (23), 83–86.

Ridge, K. W., Jenkins, D. B., Noyce, P. R. & Barber, N.D. (1995) Medication errors during hospital drug rounds. *Quality in Health Care.* **4**, 240–243.

Schelosky, L., Raffauf, C., Jendroska, K. & Poewe, W. (1995) Kava and dopamine antagonism. *Journal of Neurology, Neurosurgery and Psychiatry.* **58**, 639–640.

Schmidt, K. (1998) Just for you. *New Scientist.* **160**, 32–36.

Schulmeister, L. (1999) Chemotherapy medication errors: descriptions, severity, and contributing factors. *Oncology Nursing Forum.* **26**, 1033–1042.

Scott, G. (1997) Do antibiotic policies have an effect? *Journal of Hospital Infection.* **36** (2), 86–88.

Taylor, D. (1999) Iatrogenic drug dependence – a problem in intensive care? *Intensive Critical Care Nursing.* **15**, 95–100.

Taxis, K. Dean, B. S. & Barber, N.D. (1998) Hospital drug distribution systems in the UK and Germany – a study of medication errors. *Pharmacy World and Science.* **21**, 25–31.

Thomas, E. J. & Brennan, T. A. (2000) Incidence and types of preventable adverse events in elderly patients: population based review of medical records. *British Medical Journal.* **320**, 741–744.

Truman, P. (2000) It doesn't add up. *Nursing Standard.* **14** (43), 20.

Vale, S. (1998) Subarachnoid haemorrhage associated with ginkgo biloba. *The Lancet.* **352**, 36.

Vickers, A. & Zollman, C. (1999) ABC of complementary medicine: herbal medicine. *British Medical Journal.* **319**, 1050–1053.

UKCC (1986) *Project 2000: A new preparation for practice.* United Kingdom Central Council for Nursing, Midwifery and Health Visiting, London.

WHO (1966) *International Drug Monitoring: The role of the hospital.* Technical Report Series No. 425. World Health Organisation Geneva.

Wright, A. L. & Morgan, W. J. (1990) On the creation of 'problem' patients. *Social Science and Medicine.* **30**, 951–959.

# 6. Shifts in the Care of Hyperactive Children

*Ponnusamy Ganeson and Uttom Chowdhury*

## Introduction

The main consequence of labelling children with difficulties and problems with attention, sitting still and poor impulse control as having a 'disorder', is that a group of symptoms becomes a 'definitive' bona fide case for treatment. The controversial debate around Attention Deficit Hyperactivity Disorder (ADHD) amongst child health care professionals is, perhaps sadly, no longer dominated by challenges to the existence of ADHD, but rather the most appropriate treatment interventions to be undertaken.

The biomedical model within child, adolescent and adult psychiatry argues that illnesses such as ADHD are due to biochemical imbalances which, by logical deduction, can be corrected by medication. In this chapter, we aim to challenge this viewpoint with its reliance on universal assumptions regarding pathology and treatment and consider the possible long-term iatrogenic consequences of such a standpoint. We aim to give an overview of current understandings of ADHD from a biomedical viewpoint and explore a range of support options for families who have to deal with children displaying such behaviours. We highlight the controversy surrounding issues such as labelling, the psychosocial aspects of the 'disorder' and the use of medication. We challenge the overriding use of medication and highlight the risks that reside within such dogma. In the final section we present our recommendations.

## Background

The predominant notion of ADHD as a 'diagnosis' within the biomedical model, fuelled by powerful professionals and agencies

(e.g. health care professionals, education and not least pharmaceutical giants and the media), exerts an enormous influence. It
serves to 'inform' the lay public to the existence of a 'disorder'
which then requires 'expert' medical interventions in order to be
treated. When such perspectives become the starting point,
psychosocial factors appear to take on a peripheral role. However,
there is evidence that psychosocial factors play a crucial role in the
framework of children diagnosed with ADHD (Woodward *et al.*,
1998). And yet the case for medicating children as the first line
order of treatment has gone from strength to strength on the basis
of scientific 'facts' highlighted by research based on notions of
universal truths and objective data.

At a academic meeting held in York in October 2001, preliminary
data were presented showing that annual prescriptions of stimulants in the UK had risen from about 10,000 per million children in
1995 to almost 150,000 per million children in 1999. However, in the
case of ADHD, presumptions of universality are open to challenge
when considering the apparent cultural (Stern *et al.*, 1990) and
gender specific nature of the phenomena – it affects boys more than
girls (Dulcan, 1997).

There appears no doubt that parents and school staff feel that
they struggle daily to maintain control and motivate some children to attend to academic tasks and adhere to behavioural
norms. But children can and do exhibit defiant, oppositional
and general disruptive behaviours across a wide spectrum of contexts that one can argue to be within normal limits. They can
exhibit behaviour labelled as 'hyper' for a variety of reasons
ranging from over- and understimulation, allergies, traumas and
abuse past and present, as well as a variety of parental, family
and social dynamics. The presiding process that labels such
behaviours as ADHD appears to bypass complex psychosocial
matrices to posit a 'quick-fix', simplistic view which is readily
accepted by a population seeking relief from trying and tiring
issues. However, such processes are disempowering. As Double
contends:

'The view that the phenomena of human existence can be
understood in exclusively biological terms is obviously attractive.
If psychopathology equals bodily dysfunction, aberrant behaviour and experience can be fixed in a natural substrate.
Accountability for personal misfortune is shifted away from
personal agency and the impact of relationships. The complexities of meaning are apparently made simple. Reducing relations

between people to objective connections seems to make them more manageable.'

Double, 2001 p. 28

## What is ADHD?

Although the term ADHD is widely used amongst the public and professionals in the United Kingdom and the rest of Europe, strictly speaking the term is derived from an American classification and not from the official classification used in the UK. The fourth edition of the *Diagnostic and Statistical Manual of Mental Disorders* (DSM IV), specifies the criteria by which all mental disorders are to be diagnosed in North America (American Psychiatric Association, 2000). ADHD is a category within this classification and is diagnosed by the presence of symptoms of hyperactivity and inattention that last for at least six months. The following is a guideline for diagnosis taken from DSM IV.

'ADHD
A. Either (1) or (2):
(1)   six (or more) of the following symptoms of inattention have persisted for at least 6 months to a degree that is maladaptive and inconsistent with developmental level:

*Inattention*
   a)   Often fails to give close attention to details or makes careless mistakes in schoolwork, work, or other activities.
   b)   Often has difficulty sustaining attention in tasks or play activities.
   c)   Often does not seem to listen when being spoken to directly.
   d)   Often does not follow through on instructions and fails to finish schoolwork, chores, or duties in the workplace.
   e)   Often has difficulty organising tasks and activities.
   f)   Often avoids, dislikes, or is reluctant to engage in tasks that require sustained mental effort (such as schoolwork or homework).
   g)   Often loses things necessary for tasks or activities (e.g. toys, school assignments, pencils, books or tools).
   h)   Is often easily distracted by extraneous stimuli.
   i)   Is often forgetful in daily activities.
(2)   six or more of the following symptoms of hyperactivity–impulsivity have persisted for at least 6 months to a degree

that is maladaptive and inconsistent with developmental level:

*Hyperactivity*
  a) Often fidgets with hands or feet or squirms in seat.
  b) Often leaves seat in classroom or in other situations in which remaining seated is expected.
  c) Often runs about or climbs excessively in situations in which it is inappropriate (in adolescents or adults, may be limited to subjective feelings of restlessness).
  d) Often has difficulty playing or engaging in leisure activities quietly.
  e) Is often "on the go" or often acts as if "driven by a motor".
  f) Often talks excessively.

*Impulsivity*
  g) Often blurts out answers before questions have been completed.
  h) Often has difficulty awaiting turn.
  i) Often interrupts or intrudes on others (e.g. butts into conversations or games).
  B. Some hyperactive-impulsive or inattentive symptoms that caused immediate impairment were present before 7 years.
  C. Some impairment from the symptoms is present in two or more settings (e.g. at school and at home).
  D. There must be clear evidence of clinically significant impairment in social, academic, or occupational functioning.'

(American Psychiatric Association, 2000, p. 92. Reprinted with permission from the Diagnostic and Statistical Manual of Mental Disorders, fourth edition, text revision. Copyright 2000 American Psychiatric Association.)

If one looks solely at the diagnostic criteria, the reader might be forgiven if he or she recognises some of the symptoms in him/herself! The descriptions are normal behavioural traits in many unaffected people. In fact many health care professionals who talk about inattention will not be able to give an estimate of sustained attention for normal development.

Another criticism of the criteria is the use of the words 'significant impairment'. What does this mean? Can this be measured? The identification of behavioural symptoms and evaluation of 'impairment' is likely to be subjective and thus unreliable since so much will depend on the values and expectations of the person making the diagnosis. Thus one should not be surprised at the fact that prevalence rates of ADHD vary across centres or countries (Epstein *et al.*, 1998; Reid *et al.*, 1998). A way to limit subjective variation is to use behaviour rating scales. There are several rating scales currently in use but all still rely on subjective measures. Also, there is no sharp cut off for the diagnosis, i.e. when does normal fidgeting become a fidgeting related to ADHD? As yet, there is no general agreement on an objective measure of behaviour. We shall return to the theme of subjectivity later in the chapter.

A criticism, which is often the case in general psychiatric disorders, is that the diagnosis merely identifies a collection of symptoms and does not identify a cause of the disorder. In ADHD, some neuroimaging studies have produced interesting findings such as patients with ADHD demonstrating reduced metabolism in the frontal lobes and striatal regions of the brain (Lou *et al.*, 1984; Zametkin *et al.*, 1990). However, these findings have not been replicated in all studies.

## Labelling

Labelling a child as suffering from ADHD is to decide that there is a problem with his or her condition, and to indicate that something should be done to stop it if possible. However, once a label is applied it can potentially be damaging. As with other controversial cases throughout history, such as women who give birth out of wedlock, homosexuality, and personality disorders, does labelling demonstrate the public's intolerance of people's distinctive traits and differences from the norm?

Many critics of the ADHD label argue that it is normal for boys to be energetic and have short attention spans. By making hyperactivity an illness are we giving the medical and educational establishments more power over the lives of children? There is also the possibility of a negative effect on the self-esteem of the child who may behave in a different way as a result of the label. It must be strange being a child and being told you have a disorder that affects your abilities to concentrate and sit still. Often little thought is given to telling the child he/she has ADHD and the impact this might have on their concept of self. Nevertheless it is also not uncommon to hear of children being denied resources in school until a firm label is established. Also a label may help families move on from their perceived difficulties and learn to cope and adapt to their child's new diagnosis. Thus there are pros and cons with using the label and caution is recommended when applying such labels.

## *If ADHD does exist, what current interventions are on offer?*

Assuming other differential and competing diagnoses have been ruled out (for example conduct disorder, disinhibited attachment disorder, agitated depression etc, which may themselves be subject to criticism that they are little more than labels) what can we offer the child?

The National Institute for Clinical Excellence (NICE) guidelines for health care practitioners (NICE, 2000) clearly state that medication, if deemed necessary, should be prescribed as part of a comprehensive package. However, this is not cost-effective to the system in terms of staff and time and thus most child and adolescent mental health services and community paediatric departments will not have access to these services. Again, one wonders whether there is another agenda for promotion and advertisement of medication, sponsored by the major drug companies. Good evidence of this occurs in other psychiatric specialities. For example, there is evidence that using therapies to bring down high stress in schizophrenia is effective in preventing relapse (Goldstein *et al.*, 1978) and that family therapy is effective in helping patients with anorexia nervosa (Eisler *et al.*, 1997). Most psychiatrists know of these two effective interventions, yet the availability of these specialist mental health services is limited. The possible range of options available to support these families and their children are now explored.

### Medication

The variability of treatment and concerns about overuse of stimulants has led to the writing of clinical guidelines, and reviews of available evidence (Dulcan *et al.*, 1997; Joughin & Zwi, 1999). Prescriptions for medication for ADHD in the UK rose from 183,000 in 1991 to 1.58 million in 1995 (OST, 1997). As mentioned earlier, preliminary data show that annual prescriptions of stimulants in the UK had risen from about 10,000 per million children in 1995 to almost 150,000 per million children in 1999. Thus there is no doubt that the number of children taking stimulant medication is increasing. The use of stimulant medication varies worldwide and it is estimated to be 30 times as high in North America as in the UK (Taylor, 1999).

There are three types of medicines that are prescribed for children

112

with ADHD: *psychostimulants, clonidine* and *tricyclic antidepressants.*
By far the commonest in use are the psychostimulants. Until
recently there were three available stimulants: methylphenidate
(Ritalin), dexamphetamine and pemoline. Pemoline was with-
drawn in 1997 because of very serious concerns about the risk of
liver damage. Despite this, it can still be prescribed on a named-
patient basis by direct application to the distributors in the UK. The
stimulants are thought to work by interacting with catecholamin-
ergic neurones in the brain. However, it should be stated that it is
really not that clear how the stimulants exert their effect at the
receptor level although there have been several hypotheses put
forward in the literature. Here lies a potential ethical problem for
clinicians. Despite the fact that methylphenidate may reduce
hyperactivity and hence distress in a child with ADHD, should we
really be giving medicines to children if we do not know how they
actually work? Furthermore, are parents told of this lack of precise
knowledge of drug mechanism before they agree for their child to
take the tablets? Clearly more research is needed in this area.

The efficacy of the drug needs to be considered. There is no
doubt that stimulants can bring about a reduction in symptoms of
ADHD (Dulcan, 1997). However, the effects of medication are not
universal. Studies have shown that 75% of children with ADHD
show normalisation of inattention, hyperactivity and impulsivity
when treated with stimulants. It is not possible to predict with
certainty who will show a good response. There are too few
studies so far for settled conclusions and their interpretation is not
simple. The effects of drugs are complex and there are probably
multiple actions, on cognition and social behaviour as well as on
hyperactivity itself.

All medicines will have some form of side effects. The main side
effects include insomnia, growth retardation, and exacerbation of
tics, anorexia, convulsions and night terrors. Hence one cannot say
that stimulants are perfectly safe. Nevertheless, recent guidelines
for good practice (NICE, 2000) emphasise the need for clinicians to
monitor for side effects, yet one wonders how often this is done.
Good practice would suggest that all specialist ADHD clinics
should audit this aspect. Parents should be told of the side effects so
that they can make an informed decision on whether or not their
child should be put on the drug.

One of the presenting complaints that parents describe about
their child with ADHD is the fact that their child cannot get off to
sleep or is 'restless'. Prescribing a medication that may bring about
insomnia is counterproductive and hence it is recommended that

stimulant medicines are not prescribed too late in the afternoon or evening.

Another serious concern is long-term side effects. Again this is an area which is under-researched. The brain is not fully developed until late adolescence and thus it is not inconceivable that the regular consumption of a psychostimulant during this period may have an effect on other chemical interactions within the brain. These may not necessarily be related to physical health but there may be long-term effects on cognition or personality. One issue that guidelines and textbooks on ADHD often omit is the fact that stimulants are a controlled drug and thus there is a potential for adults to abuse the medication prescribed for their children and sell the drug on the black market.

It is interesting to consider what it is like for the child to take medication. Doctors are often too busy to ask questions related to this but it is good practice for the child to be able to have some say in whether he or she takes medication. In the UK, the current stimulant medicines are short acting, hence the child will often need to take a lunchtime tablet. This is potentially a tricky situation for the child since the child with ADHD may wish to keep the fact that he takes tablets private from his school friends. It is not uncommon to hear that some children have been teased as a result of taking 'mental' tablets within school. An increasing concern in the USA is that medication is being prescribed merely to improve and enhance academic performance. This raises a serious ethical issue. If the child has managed to improve his exam results then another parent may wish his/her child to improve academic results by taking stimulants. This is a worrying scenario as criteria other than the child's health are influencing the prescription of medication.

In the wake of controversy surrounding the use of methylphenidate to treat ADHD in the UK, NICE produced a document (NICE, 2000) offering guidance to professionals dealing with ADHD. Although the document has a few minor flaws (such as not defining what is meant by 'severe' ADHD, and making no mention of the progress of the condition and guidelines for adulthood), many clinicians welcomed the report as it emphasised the need for careful assessment and monitoring of patients on medication. Some of the issues mentioned above concerning the need to be aware of side effects were highlighted. Some critics have argued that this document is too prescriptive and has moved the issue of ADHD from the health arena to the political arena in terms of issues related to clinical governance and 'good practice'. This may be so but the document is meant to be a guide and clearly states that 'the guidance does not override the individual responsibility of health professionals to make appropriate decisions in the circumstances of the individual patient, in consultation with the patient and/or guardian or carer' (NICE, 2000 p. 1).

As mentioned in the opening of the chapter, the prescribing of medication for ADHD has continued to increase in the UK (OST, 1997). The culture of 'evidence-based practice' means that greater emphasis will be based on treatment that has been published in the medical and scientific literature as part of research and controlled trials. This should be encouraged since our patients should not be exposed to interventions that are proven to be ineffective or worse still, cause harm. Unfortunately, there is a bias here since there are more likely to be studies and trials looking at medication than there are of other treatments. This is partly because some non-drug treatment options are difficult to quantify and measure and do not lend themselves easily to clinical research studies. They may also be more difficult to carry out when it comes to controlling for variables. They are also more time consuming, hence there is also a resource implication. Research needs funding and often drug companies provide the revenue. Obviously it is in the drug companies' interests to fund research promoting their product, not to mention the amount spent on advertising the product. This reflects both their determination to sell the product and is an indication of the amount of money made through sales.

Non-drug treatment studies therefore start off at a disadvantage in the world of evidence-based practice. This does not mean to say they are ineffective. In an ideal world, there would be time and money to carry out research on all available treatment options. What then are the other available options?

## Non-drug interventions

At a recent local forum to discuss multi-agency services for ADHD, the mother of a child with ADHD made an interesting analogy: 'When patients break their hips, they get physiotherapy as well as painkillers to enable the patient to make a quick recovery. Why is it that there are so few non-drug interventions being offered alongside medication?' It makes sense that even if medication is offered, it is unlikely to sort out all the difficulties. The child still has to learn about his/her actions and take responsibility, otherwise how will he/she learn? Methylphenidate medication only lasts for four hours before it is fully metabolised and because of the side effect of insomnia, the patient cannot take the medication in the evenings. Thus even if the medication was effective, the child will still have difficulties when the medicine has worn off in the evenings. It is not definitely known that stimulant medication will lead to a better psychological outcome in the long term. Parents may not want their child to take medication because of their views and beliefs. They have a right to receive other packages of care, otherwise we are saying that we only provide help to people who accept our medicines. Medicines are said to be effective in 75% of cases (DuPaul & Rapport, 1993). Thus there will still be 25% who do not benefit from medicines and will need some form of intervention. We believe that services should develop more non-drug interventions for children with ADHD.

## Behaviour modification

Behavioural treatment takes many forms and can be focused on the child, parents, teachers, or peer group. Several trials and case studies have suggested that the approach has produced good results, especially when parents or teachers are taught to apply the skills of behaviour modification to control aggressive or severely noncompliant behaviour (Yule, 1986; Pelham *et al.*, 1993). The value of an intensive programme of psychological treatment was recently compared with medication in a major multicentre trial organised by the National Institute of Mental Health in the USA (MTA Cooperative Group, 1999). The main outcome was that a carefully executed regimen of medication management is superior to alternative treatments and is nearly as good as combined treatments. There has been considerable worldwide publicity related to this impressive study, primarily because the study was so detailed, the treatment regimen was delivered consistently across sites for many cases and numbers used were large enough for robust conclusions. However, as Taylor (1999) has pointed out, many clinicians have already misinterpreted the results as indicating a lack of effect of all intensive psychological intervention. As well as a few design factors that need to be considered when looking more closely at the trial (Taylor, 1999), the psychological interventions did not cover treatment of other potential disabling aspects of the condition such as social skills, parent–child relationship and self-esteem.

## Parent training

Parent behaviour modification training packages, based on social learning theory, have been developed for parents of non-compliant, oppositional, and aggressive children (Barkley, 1990). Parent training is a way of improving the social functioning of children with ADHD by teaching parents to recognise the importance of peer relationships, to use naturally occurring opportunities to teach social skills and self-evaluation, to take an active role in organising the child's social life, and to facilitate consistency among the adults in the child's environment (Cousins & Weiss, 1993). This form of training is relatively harmless for the child and uses simple techniques. It can also be administered in a group format to several parents at a time and thus reduce waiting lists. This would mean parents getting help at an early stage. However, despite the above advantages, parent training groups are rarely provided by community services.

## Family therapy

Family therapy may be indicated to address family dysfunction stemming either from the difficulty of raising and managing an ADHD child or from parental or marital pathology. Although there are no systematic clinical trials in ADHD, data on treatment of children with other disruptive behaviour disorders (Dadds *et al.*, 1987) and clinical experience suggest this modality as an adjunctive treatment or to facilitate consistent implementation of medication or behaviour management. This form of therapy may be useful for the child as it addresses issues with each member of the household and thus takes the 'spotlight' away from the child with ADHD, which may come as a relief for him or her. Recent research has also indicated that siblings of children with ADHD often have psychological needs which are rarely addressed (Kendall, 1999) and thus a family approach should potentially go towards meeting siblings' needs. Unfortunately the family, as opposed to the child, may be labelled as a problem through this sort of intervention.

## Training the teachers

It is important to educate teachers about the causes and treatments of hyperactive behaviour. Children may sometimes be blamed for their problems and teachers may need guidance here from health professionals. There are a number of simple behavioural techniques that teachers could use in the classroom to help the child with attention and hyperactivity problems. Positive reinforcement for good behaviour combined with negative responses such as verbal reprimands and time-out for unwanted behaviour can be effective. Rearranging of the classroom can be beneficial. For example, position the hyperactive child close to the teacher, near the blackboard and away from other similar children. This not only reduces distractions from other children but also gives the teacher a better opportunity to monitor behaviour and give frequent positive feedback.

## Nutrition

Although there is no good evidence that strict exclusion diets are beneficial in the majority of children with ADHD, some studies have shown that children may benefit from avoiding some types of food (Carter *et al.*, 1993). Parents often say they have noticed certain foods can make things worse such as cows' milk, wheat flour, citrus fruits, and food dyes. Although some parents feel that their child's behaviour may deteriorate after the ingestion of sugar, controlled studies have been unable to demonstrate any specific effect on hyperactivity (Wender & Solanto, 1991).

## Other strategies

The above are particular schools of treatment, but it is equally important to instil basic coping skills that will help the child develop and become more resilient. For instance, teaching the child certain strategies to help him or her take more responsibility by encouraging contributions, or teach decision making and problem solving skills that reinforce discipline. The child should also learn how to deal with mistakes or when things go wrong. If this is done in an encouraging and safe environment with positive feedback then surely the child will be better equipped to deal with life's day to day problems.

## *Is intervention always needed?*

One may look upon ADHD as being at one end of a normal distribution curve for general hyperactivity or impulsivity, and the children at the very extreme of this spectrum will probably have some difficulty dealing with everyday life in a mainstream school when compared to their siblings. If these children are not helped then it is likely that they may encounter problems later in life (Barkley, 1990), with underachieving, poor work records and more antisocial behaviour than controls. However, there needs to be more research in this area. The debate around diagnosis and treatment is not focused on those at the extreme of the curve but rather in the 'grey' area between 'normal' and 'disorder'. Even if the child fits the criteria for ADHD, does he or she really need intervention? Each case should be looked at on an individual basis to decide whether there is a need for intervention. This should be done involving child, parent, clinician, teachers and all professionals working with the child. Some people have even said that medication and behavioural intervention will limit creativity. People in the past who have been thought to display traits of ADHD include Thomas Edison and Benjamin Franklin.

## Other issues

The education system in the UK plays a pivotal role in raising the issue of how we as a society manage and control our children's behaviours. Our schools and educators work in difficult conditions with finite resources and often poor student–teacher ratios. This can place significant strain on teachers who come under increasing bureaucratic pressure to produce results, and who are increasingly vocal with regard to the problems they encounter in controlling and managing behaviours in the classroom. The paucity of individualised educational programmes is a logical consequence of such pressures (Maher, 2001b). In such scenarios, it can be argued that a diagnosis of ADHD offers a way out. Disruptive, inattentive behaviour can be redefined as a clinical problem rather than an educational one. Medicating a child offers a solution to the disruption caused by seemingly problem behaviour as well as absolving the teacher of responsibility related to their own coping skills and the lack of deeper holding skills within the school milieu (Hinton & Wolpert, 1998). It can be argued that the use of medication within this context serves a social control function by keeping 'problem' children docile and compliant. Often a referral for a diagnosis of ADHD is more of a reflection on the scarcity of educational psychology services that might have acted as a filter to exclude inappropriate referrals and to act as a resource for educationalists attempting to deal with pupils' persistently disruptive behaviours without resorting to the use of psychiatric services.

It is tragic that children as young as seven may be labelled with the long-term stigma of having a 'psychiatric disorder' and the risks associated with medication. Moreover, the labelling of disruptive, challenging behaviours as ADHD clearly locates the problem within the individual child, diluting the contributions of the educational system, broader family and societal environment. It may be argued that if such apparently 'disruptive/disordered' children did not have to attend school, the rate of ADHD diagnosis would drop dramatically. The level of diagnosis is perhaps a product of the need for schools to have a diagnostic label. Once this is fixed then arguments for appropriate (for someone labelled with ADHD) provision and support can be made.

Research has shown that symptoms of ADHD are often associated with relational issues such as marital disharmony (Brandon, 1971), maternal depression (Nigg & Hinshaw, 1998), critical parenting and limited parenting skills (Taylor *et al.*, 1991), hostile child–parent relationships (Barkley, 1977; Barkley *et al.*, 1983) and family

119

dysfunction (Gillberg *et al.*, 1983). However, it is of note that within such research, conclusions reached seem to lean towards a 'linear model' that suggests that it is the disorder of ADHD seated within the child itself that causes family disruption such as marital disharmony and even maternal depression. But is it not possible that family disruption itself can adversely affect a child's self-esteem, impulse control and general irritability, leading to the exhibition of behaviours associated with ADHD? Research indicates that there is a clear relationship between the behaviours of parents *towards* each other and the rate of disturbance within the child (Graham *et al.*, 1999). For example, studies indicate a link between hostility, criticism, quarrelling, remoteness and lack of mutual satisfaction within the relationship of parents and a higher incidence of 'disturbed' behaviours in children of such partnerships. Moreover, the children of divorced parents exhibit a higher rate of disturbance than children separated by the death of a parent.

The essence of the argument is that it is the parental disharmony that precipitates the dysfunction within the child, not the separation from the parent (Hetherington *et al.*, 1982; van Eerdewegh *et al.*, 1985). A discerning question to be posed would be, if the causal relationship between ADHD and disrupted families is deemed to be linear – how has such a cause–effect relationship come to be defined? We argue that the locus of pathology should not be sited within a child who has the *least* control of its family and social environment. We as health professionals must be careful that we do not contribute to the possibility of the child becoming the scapegoat for difficulties within the family.

If one is required to look at alternative causal factors for the apparent ADHD phenomena among young males, it is certainly within the family and the early socialisation of our children that the net must initially be cast. We suggest that the apparent gender specificity of ADHD as a construct is rooted in the differential socialisation of males and females and the gendered preconceptions of 'acceptable' male and female behaviours. Some 83% of children presenting with the type of disruptive, hostile, inattentive behaviours that are perceived as ADHD were male (Wolpert *et al.*, 1999). Moreover, research indicates that males are more likely to exhibit such behaviours within the school environment (Mitsos & Browne, 1998). However, these very behaviours may be considered to be merely an extension of a continuum of core constructs of maleness as competitive, oppositional, heterosexual 'machismo' (Connell, 1987; Maynard, 1993). Such constructs are invariably emphasised throughout both male and female social experiences by a media that conversely positions females as 'sex symbols, domestic drudges or virulent harridans' (Marshment, 1993). Is it any wonder that authority figures such as female teachers, who outnumber male teachers within the primary sector by some 6:1 (Maher, 2001a), vocalise experiences of hostility, denigration, devaluing and disrespect from young males seeking to live up to core patriarchal masculine identities.

Health care professionals unintentionally collude within this scenario to create diagnoses that influence how parents and teachers view the nature of children's behaviours. They contribute to the pathologising of behaviours that adults find frustrating and disruptive and, therefore, conflicts between children and adults are redefined as disorders within the children. This neatly encapsulates a spectrum of 'difficult to treat' behaviours into treatable entities. This has the added 'bonuses' of presenting such professionals as 'experts' and the opportunity for struggling adults, parents and educationalists to relinquish responsibility for their role within the dynamic.

Finally, when considering the discrepancies between referrals received from ethnic minority groups, it becomes apparent that the ADHD as a construct may also be influenced by cultural factors such as the greater focus of personal responsibility, family respectability, family closeness and the notion of 'protective' parenting within extended family systems amongst non-Europeans (Stern *et al.*, 1990). In fact the current available evidence does suggest that there may be differences in the prevalence of ADHD among nations and among racial and ethnic groups (Bird, 1996; Epstein *et al.*, 1998; Reid *et al.* 1998). Livingston (1999) describes five vignettes that illustrate cultural issues in relation to assessment of ADHD. He concludes that diagnosis and treatment will be more effective and better accepted as we get better at identifying and managing ethnocultural factors.

## Conclusion

A multiplicity of factors contribute to the conflicts and confusion in children, especially boys who are arguably trained to hide their tender sides and encouraged to be competitive, dominating and hostile especially towards women. Even if it is ultimately proven to be constitutional, the precise role of pre-natal, peri-natal and genetic factors remain unclear. Extensive literature reviews (Barkley, 1990; Hinshaw *et al.*, 1998) have concluded that family based multi-modal treatment packages can be effective for children with attentional and overactivity problems. Multi-modal programmes usually weave together parent training, family therapy, social skills, coping skills and school based behaviour programmes (Horn *et al.* 1991). Even Green and Chee (1997), who appear to subscribe exclusively to a biological model of ADHD, almost agree in principle to a multimodal treatment. However, they quickly marginalise this with the argument that this form of treatment is expensive and hard to find.

It is not only the child that has to change and learn new coping skills; the child's carers, significant adults and various guardians can assist by considering the behaviour in context and look for meanings, rather than focusing exclusively on outcomes. Those concerned with the education and training of nurses may need to open up their current focus of learning from a biomedical model, to one that includes and facilitates a broader psychosocial perspective. This may enable future nurses to take on a more proactive advocacy role on behalf of a client group that is effectively disempowered within current models.

There continues to be controversy and uncertainty about behavioural difficulties and it may be useful to consider them in multi-dimensional rather than absolutist, categorical terms. Children can be labelled with ADHD because it suits the needs of busy professionals and desperate service users. As Goodman argues: '... classifying all varieties of childhood maladjustment and distress as mental health problems is inappropriate empire building, medicalising social and educational problems that need social and educational solutions' (Goodman, 1997 p.15).

We should be concerned at the rate of increase in the use of psychostimulants such as methylphenidate (even in children below the recommended lowest age limit of six years) for our most vulnerable constituents who remain voiceless (Bramble, 1997). Within this arena, the expansion of nurse prescribing creates potential clinical ambivalence. It may be gratifying to be in a position to offer a quick panacea to those in distress, but without the broadest and inclusive perspectives as suggested here, it may be difficult for nurses not to become part of the problem instead of the solution.

The dangers are incredibly and indelibly subtle: the term ADHD is becoming common in our everyday language and thereby achieves a status of 'reality' within our experiences. Once this strand of thinking is woven into our everyday experience, we will take the predictable path of believing that 'it' actually exists. If we fail to consider ADHD with the widest of lenses and the deepest of perspectives, we will fail to help our children and their families, consigning our most vulnerable to the risk of longstanding physical, emotional and social harm.

## Reducing harm to children labelled with ADHD

> In order to minimise harm in relation to children labelled with ADHD we suggest that:
>
> i.     tighter protocols regarding diagnosis and treatment should be utilised in order to safeguard this vulnerable client group
>
> ii.    long term consideration of drug use – its appropriateness, efficacy and long term effects need to be researched and actively reviewed by *all* those working in health care
>
> iii.   attention to temperament and culture should be part of any assessment process which would attempt to place the behaviour in context
>
> iv.    good working relationships are developed between health professionals from different disciplines (e.g. joint clinics between Child and Adolescent Mental Health Services and Paediatric services)
>
> v.     liaison with schools be improved to facilitate a smoother and more coherent implementation of individualised treatment and educational programmes
>
> vi.    the intrinsic difficulties regarding diagnosis, treatment and the meaning of symptoms are shared with parents and the child
>
> vii.   those in health care should move away from a 'blame culture' towards empowering parents so they become part of the solution
>
> viii.  resources into parent education/training are increased – specifically into aspects of parenting skills that may facilitate better management of difficult behaviours and the part parents may play within this process
>
> ix.    resources within schools are enhanced improving and expanding educational psychology input to offer greater support to educationalists to help prevent and pre-empt inappropriate referrals to mental health services
>
> x.     improved training for all professional involved in the health care and education of children to increase knowledge and understanding of this modern day crisis.

# References

American Psychiatric Association (2000). *Diagnostic and Statistical Manual of Mental Disorders*, 4th edn, text revision. American Psychiatric Association, Washington, DC.

Barkley, R. A. (1977) A review of stimulant drug research with hyperactive children. *Archives of General Psychiatry*. **18**, 137–165.

Barkley, R. (1990) *Attention Deficit Hyperactivity Disorder: A handbook for diagnosis and treatment*, 2nd edn. Guilford Press, New York.

Barkley, R. A., Cunningham, C. E. & Karlsson, J. (1983) The speech of hyperactive children and their mothers: comparisons with normal children and stimulant drug effects. *Journal of Learning Disabilities*. **16**, 105–110.

Bird, H. R. (1996) Epidemiology of childhood disorders in a cross-cultural context. *Journal of Child Psychology and Psychiatry*. **37**, 35–49.

Bramble, D. (1997) Psychostimulants and British child psychiatrists. *Child Psychology and Psychiatry Review*. **2**, (4) 159–162.

Brandon, S. (1971) Overactivity in childhood. *Journal of Psychosomatic Research*. **15**, 411–415.

Carter, C. M., Urbanowicz, M., Hemsley, R., Mantilla, L., Stobel, S., Graham, P. & Taylor, E. (1993). Effects of a few food diets in ADHD. *Archives of Disease in Childhood*. **69**, 564–568.

Connell, R. W. (1987) Gender regimes and the gender order. In: *The Polity Reader in Gender Studies* (eds R. W. Connell & G. W. Dowrett), pp. 29–40. Polity Press, Cambridge.

Cousins, L. S. & Weiss, G. (1993) Parent training and social skills training for children with ADHD. *Canadian Journal of Psychiatry*. **38**, 449–457.

Dadds, M. R., Schwartz, S. & Sanders, M. R. (1987). Marital discord and treatment outcome in behavioural treatment of child conduct disorders. *Journal of Consulting Clinical Psychology*. **55**, 396–403.

Double, D. B. (2001) Can psychiatry be retrieved from a biological approach? *Journal of Critical Psychology, Counselling and Psychotherapy*. **1** (1), 28–31.

Dulcan, M. (1997) Practice parameters for the assessment and treatment of children, adolescents, and adults with attention deficit/hyperactivity disorder. *Journal of American Academy of Child and Adolescent Psychiatry*. **36**, 85–121S (supplement).

DuPaul, G. J. & Rapport, M. D. (1993) Does methylphenidate normalise the classroom performance of children with attention deficit hyperactivity disorder? *Journal of American Academy of Child and Adolescent Psychiatry*. **32**, 190–198.

Eisler, I., Dare, C., Russell, G., Szmukler, G., le Grange, D. & Dodge, E. (1997) Family and individual therapy in Anorexia Nervosa: A five year follow-up. *Archives of General Psychiatry*. **54**, 1025–1030.

Epstein, J. N., March, J. S., Conners, C. K. & Jackson, D. L. (1998) Racial differences on the Conners Teacher Rating Scale. *Journal of Abnormal Child Psychology*. **26**, 109–118.

Gillberg, C., Carlstrom, G. & Rasmussen, P. (1983) Hyperkinetic disorders in seven-year-old children with perceptual motor and attentional deficits. *Journal of Child Psychology and Psychiatry.* **24**, 233–246.

Goldstein, M. J., Rodnick, E. H., Evans, J. R., May, P. R. & Steinberg, M. (1978) Drug and family therapy in the aftercare treatment of acute schizophrenia. *Archives of General Psychiatry.* **35**, 1169–1177.

Goodman, R. (1997) Who needs child psychiatrists? *Child Psychology and Psychiatry Review.* **2**, 15–19.

Graham, P., Turk, J. & Verhulst, F. (1999) *Child Psychiatry: A developmental approach*, 3rd edn. Oxford University Press, Oxford.

Green, C. & Chee, K. (1997) *Understanding ADHD. A parent's guide to attention deficit hyperactivity disorder in children*, 2nd edn. Vermilion, London.

Hetherington, E. M., Cox, M. & Cox, R. (1982) Effects of divorce on parents and children. In: *Non-traditional families parenting & child development.* (eds M. E. Lamb & L. Erlbaum) Lawrence Erlbaum Associates, Inc. Hillsdale. 233–88.

Hinshaw, S., Klein, R. & Abikoff, H. (1998) Childhood Attention Deficit Hyperactivity Disorder: non-pharmacological and combination approaches. In: *A Guide to Treatments that Work* (eds P. Nathan & J. Gorman), pp. 26–41. Oxford University Press, New York.

Hinton, C. E. & Wolpert, M. (1998) Why is ADHD such a compelling story'. *Clinical Child Psychology and Psychiatry.* **3**, 315–317.

Horn, W., Ialongo, N., Pascoe, J., Greenberg, G., Packard, T., Lopez, M., Wagner, A. & Puttler, L. (1991) Additive effects of psychostimulants, parent training and self-control therapy with ADHD children. *Journal of the American Academy of Child and Adolescent Psychiatry.* **30**, 233–240.

Joughin, C. & Zwi, M. (1999) *The Use of Stimulants in Children with Attention Deficit Hyperactivity Disorder.* Royal College of Psychiatrists, London.

Kendall, J. (1999) Sibling accounts of attention deficit hyperactivity disorder (ADHD). *Family Process.* **38**, 117–136.

Livingston, R. (1999) Cultural issues in diagnosis and treatment of attention deficit hyperactivity disorder. *Journal of American Academy of Child and Adolescent Psychiatry.* **38**, 1591–1594.

Lou, H. C., Henriksen, L. & Bruhn, P. (1984) Focal cerebral hypoperfusion in children with dysphasia and/or ADHD. *Archives of Neurology.* **42**, 825–829.

Maher, T. (2001a) Missing men. *Young Minds Magazine.* Sept/Oct, **54**, 19.

Maher, T. (2001b) Classroom disruption getting worse. *Young Minds Magazine.* Nov/Dec, **55**, 7.

Marshment, M. (1993) Representations of women in contemporary popular culture. In: *Introducing Women's Studies* (eds D. Richardson & V. Robinson), pp. 123–150. Macmillan, London.

Maynard, M. (1993) Violence against women. In: *Introducing Women's Studies* (eds D. Richardson & V. Robinson), pp. 99–22. Macmillan, London.

Mitsos, E. & Browne, K. (1998) Gender differences in education: the under achievement of boys. *Sociology Review.* **8**, 27–31.

MTA Cooperative Group (1999). A 14-month randomised clinical trial of treatment strategies for ADHD. Multimodal treatment study of children with Attention Deficit Hyperactivity Disorder. *Archives of General Psychiatry*. **56**, 1073–86.

NICE (2000). *Guidance on the Use of Methylphenidate for ADHD*. National Institute of Clinical Excellence, London.

Nigg, J. T. & Hinshaw, S. P. (1998) Parent personality traits and psychopathology associated with anti-social behaviours in childhood attention deficit hyperactivity disorder. *Journal of Child Psychology and Psychiatry*. **39**, 145–159.

OST (1997) *Treating Problem Behaviour in Children*. Parliamentary Office of Science and Technology, London.

Pelham, W. E., Carlson, C., Sams, S. E., Vallano, G., Dixon, M. J. & Hoza, B. (1993) Separate and combined effects of methylphenidate and behaviour modification on boys with ADHD in the classroom. *Journal of Consulting and Clinical Psychology*. **61**, 506–515.

Reid, R., DuPaul, G. J. & Power, T. J. (1998) Assessing culturally different students for attention deficit hyperactivity disorder using behavioural rating scales. *Journal of Abnormal Child Psychology*. **26**, 696–698.

Stern, G., Cottrell, D. & Holmes, J. (1990) Patterns of attendance of child psychiatry outpatients with special reference to Asian families. *British Journal of Psychiatry*. **156**, 384–387.

Taylor, E., Sandberg, S., Thorley, G. & Giles, S. (1991) The epidemioilogy of childhood hyperactivity. Maudesley monograph no. 33. Oxford University Press, Oxford.

Taylor, E. (1999). Development of clinical services for ADHD. *Archives of General Psychiatry*. **56**, 1097–1099.

Van Eerdewegh, M. M., Clayton, P. J. & Van Eerdewegh, P. (1985) The bereaved child: variables influencing early psychopathology. *British Journal of Psychiatry*. **147**, 188–94.

Wender, E. H. & Solanto, M. V. (1991) Effects of sugar on aggressive and inattentive behaviour in children with attention deficit disorder with hyperactivity and normal children. *Pediatrics*. **88**, 960–966.

Woodward, L. Taylor, E. & Dowdney, L. (1998) The parenting and family functioning of children with hyperactivity. *Journal of Child Psychology and Psychiatry*. **39**, 161–168.

Wolpert, M., Hinton, C., Gardner, E., Possamai, A. & Owen, A. (1999) ADHD in the clinician audit of children with Attention Deficit and Hyperactive Disorder in the caseloads of clinical psychologists. *Clinical Psychology Forum*. August 1999, No. 130, pp. 22–26.

Yule, W. (1986) Behavioural treatments. In: *The Overactive Child* (ed. E. Taylor), pp. 219–235. Clinics in Developmental Medicine no. 97, MacKeith Press/Blackwell, Oxford.

Zametkin, A. J., Nordahl, T. E., Gross, M., King, A. C., Semple, W. E., Rumsey, J., Hamburger, S. & Cohen, R. M. (1990). Cerebral glucose metabolism in adults with hyperactivity of childhood onset. *New England Journal of Medicine*. **323**, 1361–1366.

# 7.  *The Medicalisation of Mental Health Practice – Lessons from the Care of Patients Who Deliberately Self-harm*

*Alastair McElroy*

**Editors' note**

>The author has changed parts of the cases described here to ensure the anonymity of the people, both patients and staff, referred to.

## Introduction

>This chapter explores the limits of a medicalised approach to the psychiatric care of suicidal and self-harming patients. A contrast is made between 'medical treatment', which remains largely reliant upon physical interventions, and 'psychological care' which emphasises the importance of dialogue and relationships. Implicit in the concept of a medical model is an assumption that the effects of psychological interventions are more or less innocuous because they are 'only talk'; real treatment comes from doctors and medicines. The chapter uses illustrations, drawn from the author's own research, to argue that people can be as harmed (caused pain or distress) by words as they can be by physical interventions, and that the absence of adequate nursing models allows mental health care to remain dominated by a largely inappropriate western medical culture.

## Suicide and deliberate self-harm

>Suicide remains a significant cause of death in the UK. In high-lighting this tragedy, the British government, in *Health of the Nation*

127

(DoH, 1992) and *Our Healthier Nation* (DoH, 1998), set targets for Health Authorities to introduce positive interventions and reduce the rates of suicide in the populations for which they were responsible. Unfortunately, for both users and providers of services, the relevant literature reveals an immense and complex diversity in thinking as to how this might be achieved. Theories of causation, procedures for assessment and strategies for prevention are numerous and result in a variety of theoretical frameworks and interventions being presented to those involved in suicide prevention (McElroy, 2001).

In regard to these targets, however, the role of the mental health professions is relatively unambiguous. The latter are required to provide accessible and appropriate services to individuals who, at critical times in their lives, are regarded as sufficiently distressed as to be at serious risk of deliberately harming themselves or committing suicide. The literature further indicates, however, serious problems with the role psychiatry (i.e. the medical treatment of mental disorder) plays in relation to suicide and deliberate self-harm (DSH), particularly as many individuals find the care they are offered undesirable or unhelpful (Morgan *et al.*, 1993; Sainsbury Centre for Mental Health, 1998). From a number of independently conducted investigations, it would appear that more than half of DSH patients and three quarters of suicides (Morgan *et al.*, 1993) are in medical contact shortly before their death or an episode of self-harm.

A certain proportion of 'suicidal behaviour' probably has to be regarded as unavoidable. Morgan (1994) estimated that perhaps 20% of individuals who commit suicide and 40% of those who deliberately take a non-fatal overdose, do so without giving prior warning of their intentions to friends and relatives or to medical and other caring agencies and are therefore least susceptible to preventative efforts. For some, however, 'suicidal behaviour' is foreshadowed by frequent consultations with general practitioners and the receipt of intensive psychiatric care. This population comprises a broad spectrum of individuals – from those who genuinely wish to take their own lives but have not succeeded, to those who experience quite frequent, albeit relatively innocuous, DSH episodes – for whom medical intervention would appear so far to have been unsuccessful in resolving the problems which precipitate deliberate self-harm. For want of alternatives, they are frequently admitted to acute psychiatric wards (McElroy & Sheppard, 1999), and it has been argued that the successful inpatient management of these individuals would play an important part in reducing the annual incidence of DSH and suicide (Morgan, 1994). At the beginning of the 1970s, Bagley and Greer (1971) and Kennedy (1972) suggested that inpatient psychiatric assessment and treatment did indeed have a beneficial effect on repetition. Unfortunately, subsequent studies, coupled with a re-evaluation of the extent to which inpatient psychiatric care is effective in reducing DSH, have raised doubts about the efficacy of such interventions (Sainsbury Centre for Mental Health, 1998).

Acute psychiatric wards are intended to provide intensive care and treatment for short-term episodes. There is, however, scant evidence about the effectiveness and quality of care on these wards in dealing with people with acute psychiatric problems (Sainsbury Centre for Mental Health, 1998). Relatively little is known about exactly who the people are who stay on acute psychiatric wards or what happens to them while they are there. There is a sense that hospital care is a black box, with people entering and leaving, but with little being understood of what happens in between (Rose *et al.*, 1998). The issue about quality and effectiveness of care is crucial – not least because acute inpatient treatment is the most intensive and expensive form of mental health care – but because of the worrying increase in the numbers of patients who commit suicide despite such interventions. As the overwhelming majority of hospital care is the responsibility of psychiatric nurses, part of this failure must be due to nursing procedures. The 'problem' this presents is formulated below in terms of why the traditions and practices of inpatient psychiatric nursing might be exacerbating, rather than ameliorating, the difficulties of suicidal and self-harming patients.

## The medical model and the nurse

According to Nolan (1993), psychiatric nurses are the inheritors of a role underpinned by theories and responsibilities which originate from their involvement in the management of mental illness as defined by medical doctors. Psychiatry, as a branch of medicine, operates a disease model of dysfunctioning. The methods and practices are clearly associated with the 'natural' sciences and a conviction that eventually all human behaviour can be described and understood in terms of physics and chemistry, a conviction which has come to dominate medicine. This model describes the human body as an extremely complicated physico-chemical apparatus, which functions by converting chemical into mechanical energy (Alexander & Selesnick, 1966). Using this paradigm the

129

psychiatrist largely follows the methods and procedures of the physician, looking to diagnose and treat. Accordingly, a variety of mental 'illnesses' have been associated with deliberate self-harm and suicide, with schizophrenia, personality disorders and depression being the most common (Caldwell & Gottesman, 1990).

In defining the relationship between the psychiatric nurse and the doctor, Nolan (1993) said that psychiatric nursing is regarded as part of all nursing, and the objectives of nurses working in different types of institutions will be identical, namely assisting the doctors in their efforts to cure the sick person and return them to society. There is an expectation that patients in hospital will receive some form of physical treatment – surgery and medication are the most obvious examples. The nurses in such situations will be engaged first and foremost in the provision of services that are necessary for the biological adjustment of the patient. Whilst numerous subsidiary activities are important, the emphasis is on the provision of physical care. The role of the psychiatric nurse, depending on the degree to which physical treatments for the patients are prescribed, will therefore be more or less like that of a general hospital nurse.

## Failings of the medical model

For the majority of patients who deliberately harm themselves, the rationale and implementation of this approach is problematic, and there have arisen influential opponents of the medical model. Some of the most outspoken have been self-harming patients themselves (Pembroke, 1998a; 1998b). A fundamental problem is that most medical specialities cover ground which is easy to define; this is because the speciality deals with a circumscribed part of the body (e.g. ear, nose and throat), uses a particular technique (e.g. surgery), or is concerned with a particular disease (e.g. cancer). Psychiatry, however, cannot be defined along any of these lines. Instead Eysenck (1975) believed that many psychiatrists would prefer to define psychiatry as the study of human behaviour, or as a study of interpersonal relationships, leading to a definition which leaves out all reference to medicine and redefines psychiatry as synonymous with psychology or at least a part of psychology.

A second difficulty arises from the definition of disease. If we are to recognise mental diseases, then we must have some means of knowing what a disease is, and in what ways it differs from undesirable experiences and states of being which are not diseases. Jaspers (1906, cited in Eysenck, 1975), a physician and psychiatrist, proposed that the medical notion of disease might not be relevant to most of psychiatry; in this he anticipated the anti-psychiatry psychiatrists (e.g. Szasz, 1961). Jaspers proposed the existence of three psychiatries rather than one. In the first group are those psychological or behavioural abnormalities that are based on physiological and neurological disorders of the brain and the central nervous system. Into this category would fall Alzheimer's disease and epilepsy, i.e. mental disorders due to physical processes in the brain. Jaspers's second group contains the so-called functional psychoses, i.e. mainly schizophrenia and manic depressive illness. These disorders do not manifest physical symptoms of a kind that would enable us to 'diagnose' by reference to their organic abnormality. Consequently, the notion of disease is here primarily and exclusively related to psychological and behavioural manifestations. Nevertheless a strong argument in favour of a somatic cause of these disorders is that they are now seen to respond well to certain drugs whose actions are beginning to be understood. Antipsychotic drugs certainly do truncate schizophrenic type illnesses and make recurrence less likely (Falloon *et al.*, 1985).

In Jaspers's third group there is no question of a somatic foundation or organic disease. In this group we find the majority of self-harming patients and suicidal patients who have disorders referred to as the neuroses and personality disorders. Admittedly there may be genetic factors in predisposing a person towards neurotic or 'unusual' behaviour, but these are not as specific as those involved in a psychosis. Furthermore the evidence suggests that a large number of genes are involved here, whereas in the case of a psychosis the number may be quite small (McGuffin *et al.*, 1994; Farmer & Owen, 1996). In other words, psychotic abnormality may be qualitatively different from normality, whereas neurosis, personality disorders and the other constituents of this third group are largely indicative of quantitative differences. When stress is too severe, we are all likely to suffer neurotic symptoms of some kind, or even contemplate suicide, but we are not all likely to experience schizophrenia or manic-depressive attacks. The distress an individual may feel following bereavement is a very real and potentially disabling experience, but it is hard to conceive of it as a disease or an illness. Where we are clearly not dealing with diseases but with behaviour, perhaps determined by learning, the disease concept (however defined) largely loses its meaning. It follows from Jaspers's typology that when self-harm is not attributed to a psychotic or organic disorder 'patients' will require 'psychological' rather than 'psychiatric' care.

## *Psychological care and mental health nursing*

Providing psychological care should, in principle, be foremost in the repertoire of knowledge and skills utilised by the mental health nurse. In Britain, the apparent failings of the medical model were largely responsible for a new nurse training syllabus being introduced in 1982, which unequivocally distanced the psychiatric nurse from the medical model and aimed to develop a 'psycho-therapeutic' psychiatric nurse (Nolan, 1993). The 1982 mental health nursing syllabus (no longer psychiatric nursing) for England and Wales appeared in the wake of a new philosophy which saw psychiatric hospitals as being self-evidently undesirable, an assumption often accompanied by an uncritical advocacy of community care (Weller, 1989). The apparent rejection of the medical model is evidenced by the fact that, whereas the Royal College of Psychiatrists had been consulted when previous syllabuses had been drawn up, on this occasion it was not.

This interest in the 'non-medical' contribution of the nurse in relation to the treatment of the mentally ill was not new. In 1968 a Ministry of Health report attempted to examine the present and future role of the nurse (Department of Health and Social Security, 1968). Those areas of the document that related to the psychiatric nurse appeared as opinions that were substantiated by the opinions of other writers in the USA and the UK. It was stated that:

> 'Psychiatric nurses spend much time listening to and counselling patients, or some other active psychotherapeutic role, and all carry out supportive psychotherapy to some degree.'
> Department of Health and Social Security, 1968 p. 41

However, little evidence was provided to support this statement (Cormack, 1975). Altschul (1972), for example, made an in-depth study of one aspect of psychiatric nursing when she examined the relationship between frequency and duration of one-to-one interaction between nurse and patient, and the formation of relationships. By choice she ignored all other aspects of the work of the psychiatric nurse which lay outside the one-to-one interaction. The calculations from Altschul's data revealed that only approximately 8% of accumulative time for which nurses were observed, was spent in one-to-one nurse–patient interaction, leaving 92% spent on non-interaction activities.

Importantly, and in contrast to the medical model, psychological

132

theory offers a diverse range of theory and therapeutic alternatives. As Holmes and Lindley (1989) pointed out, the activity we call therapy, as derived from psychological theory, has failed to establish itself with a degree of unity of function and purpose since its basis has no agreed theoretical foundation. Indeed, it encompasses procedures and ideologies that range from the established and conventional through to the unconventional. The full impact of this statement is made clear when it is realised that somewhere in the region of 460 diverse forms of therapy are now claimed to be in existence (Omer & London, 1988). Spinelli (1994), however, distinguished three general models or 'thematic stances' of therapy: the *psychoanalytic*, the *humanistic*, and the *cognitive–behavioural*. He suggested that together these cover the central emphasis and divergences within the great majority of theories and approaches to therapy. Even so, each of these three models has its own particular perspective on what therapy is and what it claims to offer or promote (Deurzen-Smith, 1988).

It appears, then, that doubts about the nature of psychotherapy and the psychotherapeutic role of the nurse still exist. Psychological theory does not offer a single model with which to unify the professional knowledge base but a diverse range of alternatives with the potential to create conflict and confusion. There is evidence of disparity not only between theorists and practitioners but also between practitioner and practitioner. For example, Cormack (1975) stated that whilst the need for nurses to communicate with patients was obvious, the perceived function of the communication varied from nurse to nurse. Some saw the purpose of nurse–patient communication as a diagnostic or progress measuring tool and others saw it as having a psychodynamic function. Contradictions within psychiatry are mirrored within psychiatric nursing and nurses have engaged in therapeutic practices based more on the perspective of the nurse than on the needs of the patient (Richman & Barry, 1985). Finally, the author's years of experience as a psychiatric nurse reinforce the belief that more needs to be known about what psychiatric nurses are actually doing and thinking during the process of providing psychological care to inpatients with histories of deliberate self-harm.

## Inpatient psychiatric care: models and frames

The analysis presented below is drawn from the author's own research, part of which explored the 'non-medical' management of a purposive sample of four self-harming women, aged between 20 and 40, focusing on the inpatient care they received from psychiatric professionals, in particular mental health nurses. To ensure anonymity they are referred to here as Lucy, Mary, Diane and Alice; the names of staff members have also been changed.

The empirical work referred to here was conducted on one acute psychiatric ward of 24 beds. The majority of qualified nursing staff were under 30 years of age. Professional development since qualification was limited and diverse, for example two nurses had completed a clinical teaching course, whilst another was hoping to undertake training in cognitive–behavioural therapy. None of the nurses professed any specialist knowledge, or expertise, in a particular model of care.

The aim of the study was to collaborate with nurses, doctors and patients in an effort to develop a functional and theoretically consistent framework, or model, around which to enhance the psychological care of a particular patient group. To achieve this the study emphasised the importance of reciprocity (meaning give-and-take), a negotiation of meaning and role between those involved in the research process (Lather, 1986). Laslett and Rapoport (1975) urged 'giving back' to respondents a picture of how the data are viewed, both to return something to the participants and to check descriptive and interpretative/analytic validity. The point is to provide an environment that invites participants' critical reaction to the researcher's accounts of their own and each other's thoughts and behaviours. Central to the research, therefore, was a design where respondents and researcher were actively involved in the construction and validation of meaning. The emphasis on collaboration and sharing required that 'informed consent' governed the use of data and the dissemination of outcomes. Approval to undertake the study was granted by the local research ethics committee and written consent was obtained for the verbatim responses reproduced in this chapter.

A major premise of the study was that nurses and doctors working together will differ from one another, not in whether they use a model, but in the degree to which they are aware of the model they use. As Goffman (1974) proposed, very little professional behaviour is 'atheoretical'; he contended that encounters between people are always 'framed' by a theory or belief system. Each frame offers a different perspective, the language, meaning and focus of discussions are different in each. Consequently, models will be recognisable and distinguishable from each other by the types of discourse (frames) professionals use when discussing their patients. One aim of the study was, therefore, to identify which models, or theoretical frames, were influential in determining how patient care was managed.

## The medical frame

Through an examination of the fieldnotes it is possible to identify clearly the medical frame. Here, conversations mostly concentrated on the patients' psychiatric diagnoses; their behaviours were discussed in terms of clinical symptoms that could possibly be adjusted by 'medical' prescriptions. With regard to Lucy, Mary, Diane and Alice this often concentrated on signs of depression or anxiety. The outcomes of these dialogues usually resulted in changes being made to their medication. However, there were two occasions when electro-convulsive therapy was prescribed and later administered. The medical frame did not exclusively focus on 'psychiatric' problems of this sort but included physical treatments such as inducing vomiting after overdose, suturing wounds and, on occasions, relieving constipation. Within this frame, the central activity was to define the patient's situation in biomedical terms, and to decide on the right physical intervention.

Conversations in the medical frame often involved highly technical language, expressions such as 'extra-pyramidal side effects' were common currency in discussions of the patients and their needs. Although the application of physical treatments had proven to be of limited effectiveness in alleviating the problems of these four patients, the language of the medical frame, as well as the associated skills and values, were well understood and usually accepted by the doctors and nurses involved in providing care. The patients' behaviours were discussed in a fairly detached manner and interpreted as something that need not be taken at face value, but as representations of underlying pathology. Their problems resulted from biological processes that could be identified and 'treated'. As I discuss below this was not the case when 'non-medical' frames were used to discuss patient care.

## Alternatives to the medical model

Outside of the medical frame conversations related to these patients lacked a model or theory that might have competed with these interpretations and prescriptions. Alternative opinions concerning patient care can, therefore, instead be likened to 'lay' or 'common sense' perspectives on DSH and suicidal behaviour. In other words the understanding of self-harm was, in many respects, the same to the psychiatric professionals as to 'ordinary' people – members of the public not especially involved in the management of such behaviours. For example, one psychiatrist explained aspects of Diane's personality in terms of dynamics within the family. She said:

'If you think about her family structure, [they are all] very high achieving, [for example] sister, [humanities] degree, where she [Diane] dropped out – and I am sure felt [Diane believed] that she should have been able to do all those academic things that her sister did. Dad's very upper middle class, got some flash job, you know, quite well off and I think that maybe [Diane] feels more of a failure in sort of not having achieved all of these set things like ... go to boarding school, did your degree, get a good job, and that's the sort of the pattern. I think that some people and Diane especially, being brought up in a certain way ... think that you achieve this and this in this order and you don't consider doing anything else. She [Diane] has always been so blinkered about this degree that there is no other path, there are no other options.'

In this rather confusing extract there is little, if any, technical language or theorising that would distinguish it from 'everyday' conversation and reasoning. As non-medical frames were essentially 'intuition' based dialogues of this sort they produced a variety of equivocal understandings of the patients' behaviours and divergent views on how they should be managed. There were occasions when the patient's behaviour aroused feelings of irritation or anger and stimulated the nurse or doctor's urge to be punitive rather than helpful. In the lay frames, decisions about how to respond, what to say, whether, for example, to disclose anger or to be overtly critical, were characteristically viewed as questions which related to the therapeutic stance of the individual. Nurses often expressed dissatisfaction with this and an opinion that as a 'team' they needed to adopt a collective understanding of how patients with personality disorders should be cared for. In particular, they believed that some members of staff held views regarding the management of deliberate self-harm that were incompatible with their own. The result was that in the absence of a 'psychological' or 'nursing' model the culture of the ward continued to be dominated by medical terminology and procedures (e.g. medicine rounds, ward rounds).

Importantly, as Strong (1979) has argued, an essential feature in framing (i.e. the terminology used) a situation is that the frame offers certain identities, or roles, to the participants sharing the encounter. Identities entail rights and duties, from which are derived behavioural expectations determined according to the knowledge, skills, personal attributes and status that an individual is perceived to possess. Clearly, there will be quite different reactions to opinions which emanate from a professional with presumed expert knowledge of human behaviour. From the point of view of the patient, psychiatrists and psychiatric nurses are not merely 'neutral' about mental health but are perceived to be experts. In the mind of the patient, their prescriptions and interpretations are suffused with professional judgements and evaluations. Implicit in the medical model is an assumption that the negative effects of verbal interactions are more or less innocuous because it is 'only talk' and that the real treatment comes from the physical interventions that doctors prescribe. As discussed below, however, the dialogue between patient and practitioner may actually exacerbate rather than ameliorate the problems for which help is sought and thereby cause unnecessary harm.

## Inpatient care: the patient's perspective

Over the course of the study the nursing care plans of 62 patients with self-harming behaviours (all of whom had been 'diagnosed' as having a personality disorder) were examined. With few exceptions these care plans made reference to building or forming a 'therapeutic relationship'. According to the ward philosophy, such relationships were the 'cornerstone of nursing care' and were reputedly the 'cultural norm' or guiding principle by which all staff determined their interactions with the patients. It was an expectation that staff would build or form such relationships. Primarily through interviews and observation the author consequently explored the concept of a 'therapeutic relationship' from the perspectives of Lucy, Mary, Diane and Alice, asking how they experienced the interpersonal aspects of their care, and the impact this appeared to have on their self-harming and suicidal behaviours.

Our conversations were quite wide ranging, covering most aspects of their care. The findings presented below, however, concentrate on their perceptions of the social environment, i.e. the interpersonal aspects of their care, and how this affected them. The author deliberately avoided questions that might appear to repeat the assessment procedures of the nurses and doctor and instead asked more gently and generally:

i.   What is it like being a patient here?
ii.  How do you get on with the staff?
iii. How do you get on with other patients?

Generally, as the study progressed, a gradual deterioration in relationships between the patients and staff became increasingly evident, and they had little positive to say. Alice was often inclined to be angry or resentful:

> 'This place is doing me no good, it is making me worse. I need to get out [be discharged from the ward], I need to get out. They are not offering me anything here. I asked if I could go back on to some tranquilliser tablets because I felt I needed them, they wouldn't give me them, this is why I got drunk again.'

Potentially the most damaging perception was that all four believed certain members of staff, in some cases the majority, had little time for them and that some actively disliked them. Alice said:

> 'I don't think they [the staff] like me much. Yes, like Fay [a nurse] she will ignore me, and I'll ignore her, I just don't think she likes me, but if I see Mandy [a nurse] I say hello to Mandy and she'll say hello to me. Most of the staff, they'll have a go at me for laying on the bed all day. I ignore them.'

As importantly, the patients had formed opinions of why the staff liked or disliked them. Sometimes they formed elaborate extrapolations of how they were perceived by the staff based on things they heard. Lucy had overheard a care assistant:

> 'I heard Ann [a care assistant] say "What is she doing here" in a horrible way, not a nice way. She thinks that I am wasting a bed. I don't think they like me because they see me maybe as an attractive person who "what the hell is she doing, she's young what is she doing in here?" I think that's how they see me.'

An important consequence of this was that the patients behaved differently according to which members of staff were on duty. They easily differentiated between 'helpful' and 'unhelpful' members of the team. Mary told me that she would wait and see who was on a particular shift before deciding when to ask for prn (as required) medication. She usually avoided asking the male nurses as they 'can't really be bothered'. To illustrate her point she told me how she had been 'treated' by a male nurse the previous day:

> 'I went to speak to one of the nurses and Greg was in the office with the new doctor. I said I felt really upset. He said that he was talking to the doctor and one of them would come and see me in a bit, but I could tell he couldn't really be bothered. I waited until Sandy [nurse] was around [on duty] she always has time for me. I don't know why.'

The author asked if she had discussed this with Greg but she told me instead how she had deliberately avoided mentioning it:

> 'I just didn't want to talk about it. I know sometimes I have got to face my problems and everything [but] sometimes I just want to be oblivious of them [the staff]. You know what I mean?'

We must posit, therefore, that for the most part, staff were unaware of their perceived failings or how they affected the patient. Nevertheless, the perception that one member of staff disliked them could be sufficient to alter a patient's behaviour for an entire shift, particularly if the member of staff appeared to be well regarded by his or her colleagues. Diane said she was always nervous when Ann (a nursing assistant) was on duty because, not only was she 'quite unkind', but she appeared very popular with the other members of staff:

> 'She is a care assistant on the ward and she is nice if she likes you and it seems as if sometimes she likes me and sometimes she doesn't. I have been on close obs [close observations, i.e. not allowed to leave her room unaccompanied] and everything, and outside the room I hear her talking sometimes. She seems to be bitching and you know quite like arrogant. But most of the staff think she is great so I try to keep out of her way.'

## Relationships and incidents of self-harm

Superficially the patients' self-harm appeared unplanned, impulsive and undertaken in a way which invited discovery and was unlikely to result in death. The patients' reasons for these behaviours were often confused and difficult for them to articulate. Mostly they described self-harm as a means of providing temporary respite, or escape, from emotions that resulted from an upsetting encounter of some kind. Usually this was some kind of inter-personal conflict. Sometimes they referred to an upset with a family member, sometimes of a serious degree, such as a husband leaving home, though more often it was a seemingly minor event, frequently involving a member of staff or another patient. Increasingly, however, all four patients included staff behaviour in their accounts of the events that had prompted episodes of self-harm.

Drawing a simple dichotomy between episodes of self-harm which resulted from interactions with staff, and those in which they were not involved, would be potentially misleading and unhelpful. The influences that resulted in a patient self-harming were much more complex than the notion of a single event being the sole cause would suggest. Explanations must begin from the premise that the patient is already an emotionally fragile individual who is prone to 'overreact' to things that occur in the immediate social environment. In some instances, the actions of ward staff merely represented the 'last straw', compounding negative thoughts and feelings that the patient was already experiencing. For example, in describing events that led up to one particular overdose, Lucy said she had become very nervous during a period of leave:

> 'I was really nervous because like I was going to see my family again, I was going to see my brothers just like the whole thing about seeing people makes me really like nervous.'

As the leave progressed, she had become more agitated and started to drink too much. At some point her mother told her that her aunt had been 'saying horrible things' about her:

> 'I found out that my Auntie June was saying like nice things to me, but was saying horrible things about me behind my back to my brothers. I spoke to my cousin Steven about it and he just went "Pack it in Lucy", then I just blew my top and attacked my cousin Steven.'

As a result, her cousin had refused to give her a lift back to the ward and Lucy had returned late, slightly drunk and highly agitated. Apparently she was 'told off' by a member of staff for being late:

> 'I came back here and I knew what they were all thinking and I immediately got a telling off for being late back. That was it – I took the lot [tablets].'

The 'telling off' may or may not have been intended or deserved, but the example serves to illustrate how the staff became implicated in the patient's self-harming.

In contrast to the above example, Diane described a number of incidents which had minimal external influences but were largely the product of a gradual 'building up' of interventions by the staff which she regarded as insensitive and illustrating a general lack of trust and understanding. One concerned an assessment of her that had been undertaken by a member of staff who did not know her particularly well:

> 'Recently I have had a risk assessment done to see whether I can go on leave or not and one member of staff talked to me and didn't seem to believe that I would be able to go away and I guaranteed that I wouldn't self-harm for five days and it's her lack of understanding of the amount of control I have over things that hurt me quite a lot. She wasn't the best person to talk to me because she hasn't made contact with me.'

The outcome of the assessment was that Diane was not given the leave she wanted, which left her feeling distressed and misunderstood. This was later compounded when her named nurse appeared not to take her side:

> 'Melissa [the named nurse] thought that it was done properly. She said they had looked at different things I had done, like I tried to kill myself before I went into hospital and the fact that I do tend to go out and buy harmful things to hurt myself with so they listed all the risks just plain black and white.'

Finally Diane received a phone call from her mother who also agreed that she should not be allowed to go on leave. Shortly after this, Diane went to the quiet room and cut her wrist with a piece of equipment broken from a household appliance. When the author discussed this with her she said:

> 'It wasn't the whole issue of whether I went on leave or not that upset me, it was more their view of me that was upsetting me.'

Self-harm often appeared as an immediate and purely emotional response to events with little input from cognitive processes. An illustration from Mary, however, demonstrates a process of internal reasoning that progresses from her hearing a doctor remark 'Oh, why would I want to talk to you?' to the conclusion that she was worthless and should be dead:

> *Mary*: 'Well I was in my room and there was this little doctor that comes around and, I like talked to him before and I was sat in my room and I turned down the music to talk to him and he just said "Oh why would I want to talk to you?"'
> *AMc*: 'Why did that upset you so much?'
> *Mary*: 'Well, because we like talked and things before, but yesterday he had a chat with me and yesterday I was feeling really, really negative just telling him that I want to die and I am going to die and that was all there was to it and he seemed to get really angry at that and was telling me he had worked in intensive care and he has saved children's lives and he has seen children die and he was trying to get to me like that. And it just seems to me that if the doctor thinks I must be wishing this on myself – that I must be really selfish to want to kill myself – then I must be really horrible.'

This account appeared to suggest a train of thought which took Mary from what was actually said, through a series of interconnected assumptions about what this meant, to a conclusion about how she was perceived by the doctor. This is illustrated below in Fig. 7.1.

It is important to emphasise that the decision to take the overdose not only concerned Mary's reasoning but was influenced by the doctor's identity as someone with insights and opinions of particular significance. This reflects Goffman's (1974) contention that in conversation we are often seeking approval and acceptance. The impact of a verbal exchange is, therefore, related not only to the content, but also to the teller – how a person is affected by what is said or written, depends on who has spoken or written.

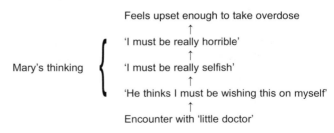

**Fig. 7.1** Self-harm following encounter with the 'little doctor'.

Staff, however, rarely examined their role in provoking self-harm. For example, on one occasion Alice attributed cutting her wrists to having drunk alcohol, and to the fact that a member of staff had criticised her for blaming other people when things went wrong:

'He [the member of staff], said to me – "It's quite handy having other people to blame isn't it?" I don't think that is very professional when you are working in psychiatry. You have kind of got to understand that everyone has got different problems.'

This particular incident was never discussed with the member of staff concerned. The entry in Alice's care plan (shown below) makes little reference to what might have been said to upset Alice. The subsequent interventions concentrate on how she could have handled the situation differently, 'challenging some of her beliefs' and reminding her of the detrimental effects of alcohol.

'A [Alice] was quite settled for the most of the morning until an incident that took place at lunchtime in the dayroom sparked A off and she became agitated and restless. It seems A [Alice] overheard a member of staff saying something she didn't like. Student nurse found A [Alice] in a heightened and aroused state having superficially cut her wrist and smelling of alcohol. She asked for time and we spent time reflecting on the harmful effects of alcohol and discussing how she could have handled it differently. A [Alice] states she doesn't want to go for weekend leave, but will try and spend time off ward whilst visiting a friend. Challenged some of her beliefs and the session ended on a positive note.' (Extract from Alice's care plan.)

'Reflecting on the incident' in effect meant considering how Alice could have behaved differently. The role of the staff member is left largely unexplored.

## New models: the role of the nurse researcher

There were strong and consistent indications that particular aspects of the social environment on the ward exacerbated the patients' problems and there appeared to be a direct causal relationship between interpersonal encounters that occurred on the ward, and incidents of DSH. Albeit subtle and unintentional, certain staff behaviours were often the immediate cause of a particular episode of self-harm. Disappointments and unmet expectations, which often went unnoticed by the staff, could assume catastrophic proportions in the minds of the four patients. This was rarely acknowledged by the team or regarded as anything more than part of the patient's problem.

Reliance on the medical model ignored the significance of relationships and undermined the importance of 'psychological' care. If what a nurse or doctor does causes unnecessary pain or distress (psychological or physical) then it is morally and professionally wrong to continue with such behaviours. This premise alone might be thought sufficient to propose the redundancy of the medical model. However, care cannot operate in a theoretical vacuum and alternative 'nursing' models, which adequately address psychological problems, have yet to be developed and evaluated.

It is a feature of 'medical' research that it emphasises a positivist methodology which deliberately distances the researcher from the population being studied. As a result, particularly with regard to in-patient care, researchers have produced descriptions (usually critical) of ward work, which are not necessarily 'owned' or understood by practising nurses. It is often unclear how the research, and researcher, affected existing values and beliefs or how the findings have been interpreted and utilised by the participants.

This is unfortunate, as every organisation, however small, has a set of beliefs and values that determine and direct its thinking and behaving. These beliefs and values create a unique culture, which is generally taken for granted by the members of the organisation (Handy, 1976). Culture will determine whether the organisation, group or profession is predisposed to change or whether it is rigid and inflexible. The culture prescribes behaviour patterns, ways of perceiving and thinking, reacting and interacting. The culture of a ward will contain beliefs about the rightness of actions and responses. Ultimately what makes it possible for nurses to function effectively with each other and to achieve their primary tasks is the consensus and acceptance of a common culture.

This study observed several different, and sometimes covert, cultures operating as different groups of staff came together on different shifts. Such beliefs and values were the currency of the 'real' culture(s), and formed unwritten sets of guidelines which practitioners followed. The written policies and procedures may have made explicit some of the ward's official norms, but a culture goes much deeper than this and the behaviour of practitioners demonstrated disparity and conflict between the 'official' culture and the actual nursing practices.

Different cultures call for differing psychological contracts (Handy, 1976), the implication being that certain types of people will be happy and successful in a certain culture and not in another. Clearly the traditions, values and assumptions about the nature of self-harm and the nurse's role will make some ways of working more acceptable than others. Inpatient care will result in confusing and negative experiences for the patients if the majority of staff do not share important beliefs and values. Nursing models are, therefore, potentially as damaging as the medical model if the subjective reasoning implicit in nurse behaviour has not first been articulated and developed into a shared understanding.

## Conclusion

One of the conclusions to be drawn from this study is that articulation, treated at length by Silverman (1997), is where a participating nurse researcher has something very important to contribute. The crucial point is that particular facets of care, e.g. frames, models or specific interventions, cannot be fully understood if they are studied in isolation from the cultures in which they operate. Instead of arguing for or against the use of a particular model or intervention, nurse researchers should investigate the values which underpin the way they are used, the circumstances that they are applied in, and the intended or unintended consequences of their use.

This would entail nurse researchers 'giving back' to participants a picture of their culture and how it appears to affect patients and staff. Argyris (1980) advocated an approach of this sort when he emphasised a re-educative or self-critical approach to social problems and practices that he felt arose from an embedded social context. Similarly, Holter and Schwartz-Barcott (1993) identified an enhancement model of action research in which the researcher's role is to facilitate practitioners in discussions of underlying problems and assumptions on a personal level as well as the level of the organisation's culture. The emphasis is on bringing to the surface the underlying value system, including norms and conflicts that may be at the core of the problems identified. Local theory emerges in such a way as to establish new cultural norms that dissipate the negative forces of competing frames. The emerging models and new theoretical insights stem from the newly formed culture. The intimacy between theory and practice that this would entail should result in the empowerment of nurses and the enhancement of nursing care offered to self-harming patients. Such models should concentrate on the interpersonal and psychological aspects of care in an effort to limit the harm caused by 'careless talk'.

## Final thoughts on models and frames

In *Asylums*, Goffman (1961) discussed the interpretative scheme offered by a total institution. An essential part was a theory of human nature, an elementary psychology used by the staff to rationalise the activities of the total institution, and to maintain social distance from the inmates and a stereotyped view of them. The use of models and the practice of power were thus closely connected. Arney and Bergen (1984) adopted the view that theories and models, by virtue of their 'professional' languages or frames, excluded some of the participants; hence all models have the effect of involving frames which exclude or disempower certain individuals and groups. In the author's own research he observed how the medical and 'lay' frames blocked communication between groups of staff and between staff and patients. The language of the medical frame in particular justified the existence of two very different and distinct identities i.e. staff and patients. Such frames have a silencing effect. An effective nursing model should invite all the participants, patients and staff, to speak to each other about their experiences. The thesis from which this chapter is drawn has at least partially developed a model of this sort, one that will create a 'common frame' and, in so doing, enhance the experience of patients who deliberately harm themselves and the nurses who are responsible for their care. It is hoped the results will encourage other nurse researchers to study the links between the worlds represented by different models and to create a dialogue between them.

## Reducing harm: issues for consideration in mental health practice

In considering limiting potential harm in mental health practice practitioners should:

i.   articulate, develop and evaluate the 'lay' models used to structure psychological nursing care
ii.  critique and evaluate the impact and value of the medical model
iii. explore obstacles to change through reflective practice, individual and group supervision
iv.  create a culture in which practitioners and researchers are partners in enhancing care
v.   involve patients and carers in all of the above.

## References

Alexander, F. & Selesnick, S. (1966) *The History of Psychiatry and Evaluation of Psychiatric Thought and practice from prehistoric times to the present.* Allen & Unwin, London.

Altschul, A. (1972) *A Study of Interactive Patterns in Acute Psychiatric Wards.* Churchill Livingstone, Edinburgh.

Argyris, C. (1980) *Inner Contradictions of Rigorous Research.* Academic Press, New York.

Arney, W. R. & Bergen, B. J. (1984) *Medicine and the Management of Living. Taming the Last Great Beast.* University of Chicago Press, Chicago and London.

Bagley, C. & Greer, S. (1971) Clinical and social predictors of repeated attempted suicide: a multivariate analysis. *British Journal of Psychiatry.* **119**, 515–521.

Caldwell, C. B. & Gottesman, I. (1990). Schizophrenics kill themselves too: a review of risk factors for suicide. *Schizophrenia Bulletin*, **16**, 571–589.

Cormack, D. (1975) A descriptive study of the work of the charge nurse in acute admission wards of psychiatric hospitals. Unpublished thesis, Dundee College of Technology.

Deurzen-Smith, E. (1988) *Existential Counselling in Practice.* Sage, London.

DHSS (1968) *Psychiatric Nursing: Today and tomorrow.* HMSO, London.

DoH (1992) *Health of the Nation: A strategy for health in England.* The Stationery Office, London.

DoH (1998) *Our Healthier Nation: A contract for health.* Department of Health and The Stationery Office, London.

Eysenck, H. J. (1975) *The Future of Psychiatry.* Methuen, London.

Falloon, I. R. H., Boyd, J. L. & McGill, C. W. (1985) Family management in the prevention of morbidity of schizophrenia. Clinical outcome of a two year longitudinal study. *Archives of Psychiatry.* **42**, 887–896.

Farmer, A. & Owen, M. J. (1996) Genomics: the next psychiatric revolution? *British Journal of Psychiatry*, **169**, 135–138.

Goffman, E. (1961) *Asylums: Essays on the social situation of mental patients and other inmates.* Doubleday, New York.

Goffman, E. (1974) *Frame Analysis: An essay on the organisation of experience.* Harvard University Press, Massachusetts.

Handy, C. (1976) *Understanding Organisations.* Penguin, London.

Holmes, J. & Lindley, R. (1989) *The Values of Psychotherapy.* Oxford University Press, Oxford.

Holter, T. & Schwarz-Barcott, M. (1993) Action research; What is it? How has it been used and how can it be used in nursing? *Journal of Advanced Nursing.* **18**, 298–304

Kennedy, P. (1972) Efficacy of a regional poisoning treatment centre in preventing further suicidal behaviour. *British Medical Journal.* **835**, 255–257.

Laslett, B. & Rapoport, B. (1975) Collaborative interviewing and interactive research. *Journal of Marriage and the Family.* **37**, 968–977.

Lather, P. (1986) Research as praxis. *Harvard Educational Review.* **56**, 257–277.

McElroy, A. (2001) Enhancing psychological nursing care, in an acute inpatient psychiatric setting, of patients who deliberately self-harm. Unpublished PhD thesis, University of Reading.

McElroy, A. & Sheppard, G. (1999) The assessment and management of self-harming patients in an Accident and Emergency department: an action research project. *Journal of Clinical Nursing.* **8**, 66–72.

McGuffin, P., Owen, M. J., O'Donovan, M. C., Thapar, A. & Gottesman, I. I. (1994) *Seminars in Psychiatric Genetics.* Gaskell, London.

Morgan, H. G. (1994) *Clinical Audit of Suicide and Other Unexpected Deaths.* NHS Management Executive, London.

Morgan, H. G., Burns-Cox, C. J., Pocock, H. & Pottle, S. (1993) Deliberate self harm: clinical and socio-economic characteristics of 368 patients. *British Journal of Psychiatry.* **127**, 564–574.

Nolan, P. (1993) *A History of Mental Health Nursing.* Chapman & Hall, London.

Omer, H. & London, P. (1988) Metamorphosis in psychotherapy: end of systems era. *Psychotherapy: Theory, Research and Practice.* **25**, 171–184.

Pembroke, L. (1998a) Self-harm: a personal story (part 1). *Mental Health Practice.* October, **2** (3), 20–24.

Pembroke, L. (1998b) Self-harm: a personal story (part 2). *Mental Health Practice.* November **2** (3), 22–24.

Richman, A. & Barry, A. (1985) More and more is less and less: The myth of psychiatric need. *British Journal of Psychiatry.* **146**, 164–168.

Rose, D., Ford, R., Lindley, P. & Gawith, L. & The KCW Mental Health Monitoring Users' Group (1998) *In Our Experience.* The Sainsbury Centre for Mental Health, London.

Sainsbury Centre for Mental Health (1998) *Acute Problems: A survey of the quality of care in acute psychiatric wards.* Sainsbury Centre for Mental Health, London.

Silverman, D. (1997) *Qualitative Research, Theory, Method and Practice.* Sage, London.

Spinelli, E. (1994) *Demystifying Therapy.* Constable, London.

Strong, P.M. (1979) *The Ceremonial Order of the Clinic. Parents, doctors and medical bureaucracies.* Routledge & Kegan Paul, London.

Szasz, T. S. (1961) *The Myth of Mental Illness: Foundations of a theory of personal conduct.* Paul B. Hoeber, New York.

Weller, M. P. I. (1989) Mental illness – who cares? *Nature.* **339**, 249–252.

# 8. Complaints as a Measure of Harm – Lessons from Community Health Councils

*Angeline Burke*

'You don't feel anything, you just feel numb. We were angry that it happened, it is just unbelievable that it can happen'

BBC News, 2001

## Introduction

Unnecessary medical harm is a concept that most people are unlikely to be able to grasp and which many would not even wish to contemplate. People go to doctors, nurses and other practitioners to be treated so that they will get better or at the very least to have their symptoms alleviated. The public take it for granted that if they are ill the health service will help them, they most certainly do not expect to be harmed by such services. Most people would accept that things might go wrong, that people may be harmed as a result and that steps are generally taken to prevent errors from re-curring. What they find difficult to accept is that a certain amount of medical harm is unnecessary and, therefore, preventable. In the example given above this was clearly the case. The quotation at the head of this chapter describes a mother's reaction following the death of her teenage son after a cancer drug was wrongly injected into his spine instead of a vein. Such is the level of trust that people place in doctors, nurses and other health care practitioners when they use the National Health Service (NHS), it is likely that the overwhelming majority would express disbelief in the same way as this mother, following a mistake that need not have happened. Since 1985, 13 similar cases have been reported in Britain. In almost all of these cases the patients died (DoH, 2000a).

149

It will be argued in this chapter that the NHS is not the most open of institutions, particularly when things go wrong and when those affected seek clarification and where appropriate an apology. In terms of seeking explanations and if necessary making a complaint, the Community Health Council (CHC) has been one avenue the public might use. Following the passing of the National Health Service Reform and Health Care Professions Act 2002, CHCs in England are due to be abolished in 2003 and replaced by a new system of patient and public involvement in health. Their successor bodies will include Patients' Forums and the Commission for Patient and Public Involvement in Health. At the time of writing (2002) the exact composition and remit of these bodies is unknown. Another part of the new system, the Patient Advice and Liaison Services (PALSs), whose function is to provide advice and support for patients who have concerns about the health service, and which are now in place (DoH, 2001d). It is clear that the aim within the Department of Health is that the public will be more closely involved and informed in future health care practice (DoH, 2002), and that they should be treated as partners by health professionals (Coulter, 2002). It is argued in this chapter that complaints, when analysed and acted upon appropriately, will remain a means through which harm in health care can be reduced. This is a position accepted by the Department of Health in the document *Building a Safer NHS for Patients* (DoH, 2001d). It is therefore worth considering the lessons learnt by the CHCs in relation to the handling of complaints.

## Complaints and the NHS complaints procedure

Complaints are made to express a level of dissatisfaction with care, treatment or the provision of NHS services generally. They may be written or verbal, formal or informal. Although complaints are not by nature positive, they are a feedback mechanism that an organisation can utilise to gain insight into user experiences. Indeed, 'Complaints provide a unique source of data for those interested in quality and risk management' (Wallace & Mulcahy, 1999 p. 59). They can be a means through which adverse health care events are first recognised (DoH, 2001d). It is important that organisations and professionals take the opportunity to learn from complaints and consider the need to change practice wherever this is necessary in an attempt to reduce errors and other forms of harm from being repeated. However, in the experience of Community Health Councils, NHS staff can often adopt defensive attitudes towards complaints and those who make them, which is not helpful in the long term. These attitudes can also lead the public to think that NHS staff in general are out to protect themselves, rather than trying to get to the root of problems there might be within the organisation. Such concerns can clearly be seen in recent government documentation on the NHS (DoH, 1999; 2000a). However, it is clear that the government wishes to see a more open NHS, one that is prepared to listen more closely to users of the service.

It is worth noting that not all dissatisfaction will result in formal complaints being made, so such complaints are only an indication of the scale of problems in the NHS. Complaints may not be made for a number of reasons. Some people do not like confrontation, some believe that making a complaint will have little or no effect, and some fear that they will be victimised if they make a complaint. For example, CHCs were aware that people have been removed from their general practitioner's (GP) list when they have made complaints.

The NHS complaints procedure consists of two stages (see Fig. 8.1). The first stage, known as *local resolution*, is designed to facilitate the answering of complaints quickly and informally. Trusts, health authorities and primary care practitioners must have procedures for dealing with complaints about their services. There is, however, a degree of flexibility in that they are able to handle complaints in any way that they believe will resolve the matter to the satisfaction of complainants.

If complainants are dissatisfied with local resolution they can ask for referral to an *independent review panel* (IRP). However, there is no automatic entitlement to a review and the decision about whether to grant one is made by a convener and an independent lay person. If a complaint is not referred to an IRP the complainant has a right to pass the matter to the *Commissioner for the Health Service*, also known as the Health Service Ombudsman (HSO). A complainant may also refer their case to the HSO if they remain dissatisfied with the way their complaint has been handled. The HSO is independent of the NHS.

The Department of Health (DoH) commissioned an evaluation of the NHS complaints procedures, as implemented in 1996, to see how they were operating and to inform their future development (York Health Economics Consortium, 2001). This evaluation concluded that, from the perspectives of complainants and those who operate the procedure, they are not working well and improvements are needed. Wallace and Mulcahy (1999) reached similar conclusions. The DoH-commissioned evaluation found that there was a high level of dissatisfaction with the procedures amongst

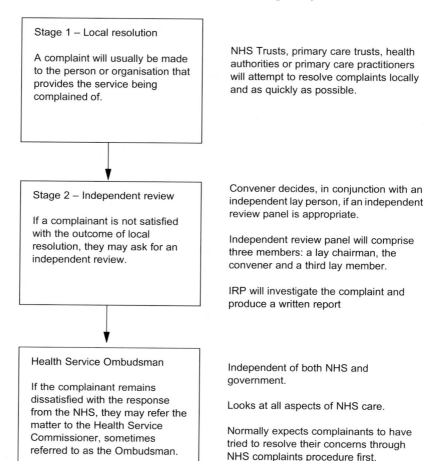

Stage 1 – Local resolution

A complaint will usually be made to the person or organisation that provides the service being complained of.

NHS Trusts, primary care trusts, health authorities or primary care practitioners will attempt to resolve complaints locally and as quickly as possible.

Stage 2 – Independent review

If a complainant is not satisfied with the outcome of local resolution, they may ask for an independent review.

Convener decides, in conjunction with an independent lay person, if an independent review panel is appropriate.

Independent review panel will comprise three members: a lay chairman, the convener and a third lay member.

IRP will investigate the complaint and produce a written report

Health Service Ombudsman

If the complainant remains dissatisfied with the response from the NHS, they may refer the matter to the Health Service Commissioner, sometimes referred to as the Ombudsman.

Independent of both NHS and government.

Looks at all aspects of NHS care.

Normally expects complainants to have tried to resolve their concerns through NHS complaints procedure first.

**Fig. 8.1** An outline of the NHS Complaints Procedure (Department of Health, 2001a).

complainants, with a significant number of them finding the process stressful. One cause of stress is likely to be the length of the process. It is not uncommon for a complaint to take 2–3 years to go through the NHS complaints procedure (York Health Economics Consortium, 2001). If complaints procedures are protracted it can hinder complainants' recovery from their experiences and it is widely accepted that stress can have an adverse effect on health. Following the evaluation of the complaints procedures (York Health Economics Consortium, 2001) the Department of Health is proposing to make changes. At the time of writing, it is not yet clear what these will be. It is important to acknowledge that complaints about deficient practice may lead to the referral of the matter to the relevant professional body. For example, complaints about nursing staff may be made to the Nursing and Midwifery Council (NMC, 2002).

## The work of Community Health Councils in supporting complainants

CHCs were perhaps best placed to understand the everyday reality of the management of complaints. This had not been their primary role, but it is clear that some patients who wished to engage NHS organisations in dialogue about particular aspects of their care, had found the need to approach these independent organisations for help and support. It could be argued that this is evidence enough that NHS organisations and practitioners are not aware of the vital role that complaints can play in quality assurance.

CHCs were established because scandals involving the abuse and neglect of patients in long-stay mental hospitals demonstrated to politicians and the public that managers and professionals had not always protected vulnerable patients in their care (Hogg, 1996). Their work and their responsibilities towards patients, somewhat inevitably, resulted in conflicts of interest. CHCs were set up under the National Health Service Act 1973 (HMSO, 1973) and came into being the following year. The National Health Service Act of 1977 and the Community Health Councils Regulations 1996 (amended in 2000) governed them. The remit of CHCs was to represent the interests of the public within the health service. In other words they were introduced to act as 'watchdogs' on behalf of the public.

There were over 200 CHCs in England and Wales with bodies performing similar functions in Scotland (Local Health Councils) and Northern Ireland (Health and Social Services Councils). They consisted of a small number of paid staff, usually two to three officers, who provided professional support to voluntary members. Together they operated from a small CHC office. Depending upon the geographical area covered by a CHC, they would have between 16 and 30 members. In 2000/01 the annual budget for CHCs in England was £22 million, which, although a significant amount of money, is a fraction of the total spending on the NHS. Although for administrative purposes CHCs received their funds from the Department of Health, they were independent, autonomous bodies. As long as they fulfilled their statutory duties and responsibilities, they were able to work as they chose within the statutory rights and duties set out below.

## Statutory rights of CHCs

Community Health Councils are endowed with the following statutory rights.

i.   Health authorities have a duty to consult their local CHC before making any decisions that would substantially change or develop health services in the area.

ii.  To refer inadequate consultation exercises about substantial changes to the Secretary of State for Health for a decision.

iii. To be consulted on any proposals to establish, merge or dissolve NHS Trusts.

iv.  To be provided with information from health authorities. Exceptions to this right include the provision of information related to personnel matters, the diagnosis and treatment of individuals and, the disclosure of information prohibited by law.

v.   To inspect premises providing NHS treatment or care. This right extends to NHS Trusts, and private sector facilities where NHS care is purchased.

vi.  Health authorities must meet with local CHCs at least once a year to discuss matters of mutual concern and interest.

## Statutory duties of CHCs

Statute imposes the following duties on CHCs. By law they:

i.   are required to keep under review the operation of the health services in their districts and advise and make recommendations to the relevant health authorities about the operation of local health services

ii.  must inform the Secretary of State for Health when they consider that consultation has not been carried out properly

iii. must hold their meetings in public at intervals of not more than three months

iv.  must produce annual reports of their activities and ensure that they are available to the public, the Secretary of State for Health and relevant health authorities and Trusts (Community Health Councils Regulations 1996, as amended).

CHCs were supported and represented at a national level by the Association of Community Health Councils for England and Wales (ACHCEW). The statutory duties of ACHCEW were to advise CHCs with respect to the performance of their functions and to represent those interests in the health service at the national level.

## Community Health Councils, primary care and the private sector

In terms of legal rights, CHCs had none in relation to primary care. They did not, for example, have a right to visit and inspect GP premises in the same way that they are able to visit and inspect NHS hospitals. They could only visit with the consent of the practitioners involved. CHCs had, however, been able to assist people who had complaints about primary care. Despite the absence of legal rights in this area many CHCs forged good 'unofficial' working relationships with primary care providers. It is important to note that the rights of CHCs did not in general extend to the private sector. A survey of CHCs (Griffith, 1997) gave a number of examples which illustrate the sorts of issues complaints can highlight. These have ranged from small improvements in local services and work on behalf of lay individuals to significant changes in health service provision.

Tameside and Glossop CHC helped to support members of the public affected by the activities of the general practitioner Harold Shipman (Baker, 2001), who was convicted of multiple murder. The CHC pushed for a judicial review of the Secretary of State's decision not to hold a public inquiry into the matter. The CHC lobbied Members of Parliament and worked with ACHCEW, putting their weight behind the case made by the relatives of the victims for a public inquiry. The review subsequently overturned the decision to hold the inquiry in private. It was hoped that the outcome of the public inquiry would offer clear and effective recommendations to protect patients in the future (Tameside & Glossop CHC, 2001).

More recently South East Kent CHC supported women who had been treated by the UK gynaecologist Rodney Ledward (Ritchie Report, 2000) and helped to expose the extent of his malpractice (see also Chapter 2). The local CHC organised a meeting of women who had been treated by Ledward and who were worried after they learned of investigations by the General Medical Council. The scale of the problem was indicated when 200 women attended the meeting. The CHC set up a database with details of individual cases and arranged meetings with patients and gynaecologists from the NHS Trust involved to help ascertain if aspects of Ledward's treatment had been inappropriate. Eventually 480 women approached the CHC on this matter. Doubts about their treatment were only triggered in some women as a result of the publicity surrounding the case. Only a handful of patients had complained about their treatment at the time and 'Many did not know how to complain or to whom to complain, many were too embarrassed to do so...' (Ritchie Report, 2000 p. 14). The CHC also found that a number of the women had been encouraged to have private treatment. This meant that complaints from this area could not be investigated under the NHS complaints procedure.

## Supporting complainants

It is essential that when things do go wrong, when patients suffer unnecessary harm or are harmed inadvertently, they have recourse to appropriate forms of redress. It was generally the experience of CHCs that most wanted little more than an apology and an assurance that mistakes would not be repeated. This is not too much to expect, but for many, as discussed earlier in this chapter, experience of the NHS complaints procedure can be distressing (York Health Economics Consortium, 2001).

Liverpool Eastern CHC supported the parents of children whose organs were removed post mortem, without consent, at Alder Hey Hospital. The following quotation illustrates the range of roles CHCs could take in supporting members of the public seeking answers to questions about the conduct of those working within the NHS. It was noted that the parents seeking answers to their many questions found it a frustrating and often unsuccessful ordeal. They felt that nobody understood their distress and did not know which way to turn.

> '... We spoke to many people in authority and though individuals gave us their sympathy, it seemed nobody could give us any advice as to how we should handle this dreadful situation. It was not until we were advised to contact [the CHC representative] ... at the CHC in Liverpool that we felt here was somebody who was actually willing to listen to us.... We were given practical advice on how to request our son's medical records and information on the forthcoming internal inquiry and how we could be part of that inquiry. We were given a sense of direction and for that we will always be grateful.'
>
> Robinson, 2001 p. 1. Reproduced with permission

Through the contact with the CHC a support group was formed called PITY II. The Chief Officer of the CHC became the secretary and her experience was invaluable in dealing with the difficult situation at Alder Hey. The parents noted that they had come to realise that the CHC plays a vital role in the community when it comes to ordinary people dealing with the NHS, helping them to break down the barriers of officialdom and cutting through red tape.

It is not currently possible to deal with complaints involving more than one part of the NHS under a single system. A single 'patient journey' as the following illustrative scenario shows could conceivably result in the need for a complainant to register a number of complaints. For example, a patient contacts her GP requesting a home visit late at night. The GP refuses to visit, an ambulance has to be called and there is a long delay before it arrives. The patient is taken to the Accident & Emergency (A&E) Department and is forced to wait for many hours in the department on a trolley before she is admitted to a ward. During her stay in hospital the patient has a number of concerns about her care and treatment. In such a case the patient would need to lodge separate complaints with her GP, the ambulance NHS Trust and the hospital NHS Trust. Each complaint could involve both local resolution, applications for investigation of the complaints by independent review panels, and investigation by the Health Service Ombudsman. It could be argued that the patient should be able to make a single complaint about all aspects of care or treatment involving the NHS. The process would become even more complicated if private health care services had been used.

Although not recognised as a statutory duty, supporting complainants had become a large and significant part of the work of CHCs. They were not specifically funded to do this work but most did it in recognition of the fact that there was need for such support. It is essential that those who need help in navigating the complaints system are able to get free, independent and confidential support.

> 'The expertise CHC officers have developed in the complexities of the complaints arrangements is important in enabling people to take forward concerns which they might have otherwise felt unable to do. People may find themselves bringing a complaint at a time of great personal stress, such as following a death or serious illness. The support of an independent advocate at such times has been identified by complainants as invaluable'
>
> Wong, 1999 p. 3

## The nature of complaints

The Government Statistical Service (DoH, 2001a) reported that during the financial year 2000/01, 95,994 written complaints were made about Hospital and Community Health Services (see Table

157

**Table 8.1**  Written NHS complaints in the financial year 2000–01 (Department of Health, 2001a).

| Total number of written complaints about hospital and community health services | | |
|---|---|---|
| *By profession* | Medical (including surgical) | 43,930 |
| | Nursing, midwifery and health visiting | 19,020 |
| | All others | 33,044 |
| | Total | **95,994** |
| *By main subject of the complaint* | All aspects of clinical treatment | 32,809 |
| | Appointments, delay/cancellations (outpatient/inpatient) | 16,550 |
| | Attitude of staff | 12,439 |
| | Communication/information to patients (written and oral) | 8,889 |
| | All others | 25,307 |
| | Total | **95,994** |
| In addition to the above 44,442 written complaints were also received with regard to family health services. | | |

8.1). Of these 43,930 were against medical staff (including surgical) and 19,020 were about nursing, midwifery and health visiting staff. In terms of the subject about which complaints were made, a total of 12,439 related to staff attitude compared with 32,809 about aspects of clinical treatment. The total number of written complaints received about family health services, in addition to those figures given above, was 44,442.

It has been estimated that CHCs assisted some 30,000 complainants each year. This is an average of 145 complaints per CHC per year (Insight Management Consulting, 1996). An analysis of the complaints work of CHCs (Ellis, 1996) found that the majority of complaints concerned inappropriate treatment/care and that around one in ten complaints concerned problems about staff attitude.

An example of a complaint is that of a family accused of child abuse by hospital staff, and who turned to a CHC for help. Following an epileptic fit their young baby was admitted to hospital. Staff suspected shaken baby syndrome. Medical records in fact showed that the problem had been caused by a haemorrhage which the hospital had failed to notice when the baby was born at the hospital. By the time the records were found (within hours of the accusation of child abuse being made) child protection proceedings had started. With the help of the local CHC the family fought for five years to clear their name and to have medical and social services records corrected. The CHC put together a case about what had happened to the family. The mother was reported in *The Times* to have said that 'The hospital told us it was out of its hands. Things changed when the CHC stepped in. Most people fall at the first hurdle. But the CHC allowed us to negotiate the hurdles because it knew the ropes and was not associated with the hospital. It kept up the drive for truth' (Crompton, 2001 p. 8).

## Disabling complainants

The Association of Community Health Councils for England and Wales became aware of an increase in the number of cases where health care staff had responded to complaints by patients and their representatives, with the threat of defamation proceedings. This prompted them to carry out a survey of CHCs to find out how common this was. A person claiming defamation must prove that they have been slandered or libelled and show that their reputation has been impugned. The report of the survey outlines ways in which the threat of proceedings for defamation is undermining the quality drive within the NHS by, for example, causing people to withdraw their complaints.

> 'One complainant made initial contact with the CHC when she received a response to her complaint about her GP. The practitioner had construed a general comment as defamatory and the tone of his letters threatening legal action, was so intimidatory that the client decided not to pursue the complaint. The situation was causing her severe emotional distress. The client felt that she was bullied into discontinuing her complaint and is still fearful of the threat of action.'
>
> Chester, 2000 p. 6

The chief executive of an NHS Trust added to the pressure felt by the complainant by writing a letter stating that if the details of the complaint were to be relayed to nursing staff they might consider taking defamation proceedings (Chester, 2000).

Such threats, and the defensive, arrogant and even aggressive behaviour sometimes encountered by the public from NHS staff when legitimate complaints are made, are disabling. They discourage the public from making complaints or make the process more traumatic than it needs to be. They also disadvantage the organisation as the situation that led to the complaint is likely to occur again.

## The NHS – *moving towards a culture of openness?*

Community Health Councils' support for complainants was not always welcomed and this may be mirrored within the system that replaces them. A survey of general practitioners looking at their experiences of patients' complaints cited a number of adverse comments relating to CHCs. They were described as trying 'to stir up trouble', 'loves picking a fight with general practitioners', 'victimise the general practitioner unduly', and 'manipulates the patient to make the complaint' (Jain & Ogden, 1999). A CHC accused a GP of refusing a patient a pregnancy test but the CHC complaint was not upheld. Following the failure of the complaint the GP tried to have the CHC investigated and to obtain an apology. Having failed to get an apology the GP took his campaign against the CHC to the European Commission of Human Rights (ECHR). The ECHR rejected the GP's complaint because it was out of time (Anon, 1991 p. 16).

Complainants have spoken about hospital staff risking their jobs to help them to pursue a complaint. Staff should not be put in a position where they have to trade off protecting patients against putting their jobs at risk. Besides, as has been shown by the inquiry into the work of the gynaecologist Rodney Ledward, not all staff are prepared to do this (Ritchie Report, 2000). It is clear from the inquiry that had staff spoken out about concerns they had about Ledward's performance, patients could have been protected from harm. The report of the inquiry states that 'It became clear very early in our investigation there was, and probably still is, a culture of junior doctors being reluctant to criticise their senior colleagues because it might jeopardise their careers, as they are so dependent on their senior colleagues for references' (Ritchie Report, 2000 p. 16).

The Ritchie Report also points out that a significant number of the nursing staff were reluctant to make contact with the inquiry and give evidence. Reasons for their reluctance fell into the following categories: many felt their views were insignificant and did not wish to criticise consultants; many were frightened about giving evidence because they felt they might be criticised for not speaking out earlier; and some were anxious that they might be disciplined by their governing body and their livelihoods might be placed in

jeopardy. The Bristol Royal Infirmary Inquiry (2001) also highlighted the need for the NHS to foster a culture of openness so that
staff can feel safe if they wish to raise and discuss issues of concern,
a change accepted by the Department of Health (DoH, 2002).

The jobs of whistleblowers, those staff that disclose information
reasonably and responsibly in the public interest, should not be put
at risk particularly where patients' lives are at stake. The NHS
should be open, honest and accountable. CHCs supported the
introduction of the Public Interest Disclosure Act 1998, which was
designed to give statutory protection to employees who disclose
information reasonably and responsibly. However, although a step
in the right direction, it may not go far enough. For example, under
the Act, health authorities and Trusts are not obliged to set up
whistleblowing policies although the Department of Health claims
that '... the Government has introduced one of the most far-
reaching whistleblower protection laws in the world to ensure that
any member of NHS staff can speak out against poor standards
without fear of victimisation' (DoH, 2001a p. 27). There is, however,
little evidence to suggest that staff will be encouraged to share their
concerns with agencies like the CHC.

The Ledward Inquiry (Ritchie Report, 2000) made a number of
recommendations about whistleblowing which, if implemented,
would facilitate greater openness in the NHS and move the organisation away from the blame culture which prevents practitioners
from raising concerns about safety and errors. This would be in the
interests of patients and staff. Above all, the public must be assured
that when things go wrong they will not be covered up.

## Beyond complaints: specific Community Health Council initiatives

As well as supporting individual complaints, CHCs were active in
identifying areas where there were potential problems. In a sense, in
these areas they are making a 'collective complaint' that reasonable
standards are not being met.

### Casualty Watch

Casualty Watch was a snapshot survey by CHCs of how long
patients wait in Accident and Emergency Departments (A&E) and
came to be a thorn in the side of many hospital staff including
managers. Casualty Watch was conducted by some CHCs on a
monthly basis, and by most annually. The Department of Health
has also measured waits in A&E departments but only recording
how long people wait on trolleys. CHCs captured the patient

experience by measuring the length of wait from the time of arrival to the time of discharge or admission to hospital. The Department has criticised the measure of the total wait saying that it is misleading because it does not take into account the fact that some patients are under observation or may, for example, be awaiting test results. However, following the Nationwide Casualty Watch (Burke & Benham, 2001), the Department conceded that the methodology used by CHCs is a better measure:

> '... we want to change the way waiting times in A&E departments are monitored. The current system measures the waiting time from the decision to admit and the time of admission to a bed. We are developing plans to replace this with a new system which measures waiting time from the point a patient arrives in A&E to admission, transfer or discharge – which will be a much better measure of patients' real experience in A&E departments.'
> DoH, 2001c p. 2

Casualty Watch is viewed by some people as not being helpful and as being an attack on overstretched staff. However, the Royal College of Nursing (RCN), instead of being defensive about the problems, recognised the value of Casualty Watch and in 2000 they worked with the Association of CHCs to carry out a joint survey. This looked at the impact of long waits on patients, staff and other hospital wards and departments. Following the survey the General Secretary of the RCN said: 'Nurses are at breaking point, concerned that they can't even provide the basics of care' (RCN, 2000 p. 1).

Patients subjected to long waits in A&E departments may find that they are harmed because they are not receiving care on an appropriate ward from appropriately trained staff. They may be harmed physically because trolleys in these departments are not designed for prolonged use by individual patients and they may also experience harm because the environment in many A&E departments is not conducive to their wellbeing. By highlighting the unacceptably long waits that people face in A&E departments, CHCs were able to bring about positive changes which in themselves have probably reduced subsequent complaints on this matter. Without the persistent scrutiny by CHCs it is likely that the problem of long waits and the causes of them would not have been addressed as a priority at a national level.

## Hungry in hospital?

A survey by CHCs of nutrition and hospital mealtimes graphically illustrated that some patients do not get enough to eat and drink (Burke, 1997). This is a clear example of everyday harm in health care. There are a number of reasons why this may happen, including the lack of clarity about who should be responsible for ensuring that patients eat and drink enough when they are in hospital, and who should be responsible for actually feeding patients. Also, in the medically influenced, treatment oriented environment of the general hospital, nutrition may not be seen as a priority. Nurses have traditionally played a key practical role in meeting the nutritional needs of hospitalised patients (RCN, 1996) and the United Kingdom Central Council stated that it should be a nurse's role to ensure that patients are fed properly, although responsibility for this could be delegated (UKCC, 1997). Clearly, however, over the years there has been a withdrawal of nursing input at mealtimes. Is this because the nursing role is expanding and nurses are now expected to carry out, or prefer to carry out what might be seen as more interesting, frequently technical tasks? It could be argued from the perspective of the patient that nurses, in their pursuit of professional goals, are neglecting the basic need of patients to be adequately nourished.

## *Expanding information technology*

Although there are clear benefits to be gained from technology in health care, and it is clear that its use will spread. A report by the Association of Community Health Councils (1999) highlights a number of possible concerns that should not be overlooked in any developments in this field. They included the following.

i.   A lack of clarity about provider responsibilities. If the service is provided at a distance, who, in the event of a complaint, would be held responsible? The 'host' clinic/surgery, hospital etc. or the site responsible for providing the consultation? This issue would be of particular importance if the link was international.

ii.  In the experience of CHCs, patients frequently experience difficulties in accessing their medical records including being asked to pay exorbitant charges for this. This problem could be exacerbated if audiovisual records are made but are not easily accessible.

iii. Without satisfactory arrangements the very advantages of computerisation, relating to ease of access, storage and pro-

cessing could severely compromise the confidentiality of patients' records (see also Williams, 1998).
iv. Patients may be denied face-to-face consultations in favour of telemedicine which may be depersonalising and patients may feel inhibited about asking questions. Health care professionals will need to be fully trained in relevant communication skills.

Similar concerns have been expressed about some aspects of NHS Direct, the nurse-led information line for the public (see Chapter 11). These initiatives may prove to be valuable tools in reducing harm in health care, but it is important that as telemedicine and NHS Direct are developed they are independently assessed. This should include input from the public as well as professionals, to ensure that any developments are proven to be in the interest of the general public rather than just being organisationally expedient.

## Limits and reform of Community Health Councils

Not all of those in authority recognised the potential of CHCs to support complainants or if they have, they have in some cases been alarmed by it or have resisted it (Commission on the NHS, 2000). In other parts of the world, particularly in Europe, the CHC model of public representation is revered. In an interview a World Health Organisation adviser observed, 'CHCs are a jewel – that is not well understood . . . There is nothing like it in the rest of Europe, where it is the administrators and doctors who decide' (Healy, 1998 p. 13). Griffith (1997) noted that a degree of criticism from NHS bodies is inevitable since it is CHCs' role to keep their activities under review and some managers and professionals are bound on occasion to find that uncomfortable. Members of the public were also, at times, less than satisfied with the service they have received from CHCs. Such dissatisfaction stemmed in part from the very limited resources available to CHCs, which sometimes limited their ability to meet the demands made of them.

Limited legal powers also created difficulties for CHCs. The NHS had seen dramatic changes since the inception of CHCs, yet their statutory powers had not kept pace with the changes. For some years now the NHS has been moving towards becoming primary care led. Yet, as mentioned earlier in this chapter, CHCs did not have any legal rights in relation to primary care. Neither did the remit of CHCs extend to private health care and so complainant support from this area was therefore limited. This is clearly un-satisfactory considering that many people are turning to private care in the UK to avoid problems in the NHS such as long waiting lists and difficulties in accessing NHS dentistry. The CHC involved in the Ledward case found that many women had been encouraged by him to have their treatment privately, something subsequently confirmed within the Ritchie Report (2000). They were unable to acquire adequate support in making complaints because they were outside the NHS.

The Department of Health is taking steps to increase private sector involvement in the NHS, believing that this will be in the interests of patients. When signing the Concordat (agreement) between the NHS and the private sector the Health Secretary said, 'Using spare capacity in the private and voluntary sector will mean more patients can be treated, more quickly' (DoH, 2000b p. 1). However, Pollock *et al*. (2001) in a briefing about health and privatisation produced prior to the general election that year, expressed concerns about these developments for a number of reasons: 'The current regulatory framework places no obligations on private hospitals to identify or to investigate significant failures in medical practice' (p. 7), and that 'The NHS has also picked up the pieces of poor private sector performance. Last year there were 142,000 admissions from private hospitals to the NHS' (p. 1). Currently there is no system in place to bridge this provision if a complaint is made.

In view of these developments it would seem essential that private patients and users of private care institutions at public expense have access to meaningful complaints procedures. Calculations in the Bristol Royal Infirmary Inquiry (2001) estimated that there were around 25,000 annual deaths in NHS hospitals from preventable adverse events. There is good reason to suppose that a proportionally comparable figure would be found if similar calculations were made on private hospital provision, and bearing in mind the evidence from the Ritchie Report (2000) levels of unnecessary harm might be higher than in the NHS.

Such a position is particularly worrying as CHCs had for years been aware of limitations in their ability to represent the public voice in the NHS and had called for reform of their statutory duties and responsibilities. But rather than strengthening and developing CHCs, in July 2000 the government put forward plans to abolish them in England. A central plank of the NHS Plan (DoH, 2000c) was to place patients at the heart of the NHS and the development of systems that would suit the needs of patients rather than systems that would suit the organisational needs of the NHS. Very few people could argue against these intentions and CHCs certainly felt that putting the needs of patients uppermost in the NHS was not before time. The proposed replacements were met with a great deal of opposition from individuals, patient and professional organisations, Members of Parliament and many others. There was a widespread consensus that CHCs should not be abolished until a system of public representation and involvement that was at least as effective as CHCs had been developed. Almost two years after the plan to abolish CHCs in England was announced, the roles and operation of their replacement bodies were finally developed and refined, leading to an acceptance in Parliament that CHCs could be abolished.

As part of the Health and Social Care Act 2001 (HMSO, 2001) an Independent Complaints Advocacy Service will be established to support people who wish to make a complaint about the NHS. This is a welcome development but how the service will work in practice has yet to be decided. Under the Act, local authorities have also been given the power to scrutinise the NHS at a local level. It should be noted, however, that this is a power, not a duty, and as such it is possible that scrutiny may not take place. Each NHS Trust and Primary Care Trust should have a Patient Advice and Liaison Service (PALS) to work with patients and their carers to resolve problems with services on the spot. Again, this customer service role is to be welcomed but concerns have been expressed because, as employees of the Trusts, PALSs may not be independent so their work in supporting patients and their carers could be compromised.

## Conclusion

This chapter, using the work of the CHC, has illustrated both the nature and incidence of complaints reporting in the NHS. Although, by the time of publication, CHCs will have gone, there are lessons to be learnt from the work they undertook. It is clear that complaints, although not always seen in a positive light by those working in the NHS, have been a window through which harm in health care, in its various guises, can be recognised. The DoH (2001d) accepts that they are a mechanism through which such goals can be achieved, but that the complaints system needs to be improved and made more open and less time consuming for the complainant.

Public confidence in the NHS has been rocked by a series of high profile scandals, such as those of Shipman (Baker, 2001), Ledward (Ritchie Report, 2000) and the Bristol Royal Infirmary

(Kennedy *et al.*, 2000; Bristol Royal Infirmary Inquiry, 2001; DoH, 2002), involving doctors, nurses and other staff and the culture of defensiveness that has come to light as a result of these scandals. That confidence needs to be restored. The NHS should be open and transparent. One way to reduce unnecessary harm is not to be defensive about complaints, but to learn from them and change practice and the systems used within practice where necessary, to prevent mistakes and other forms of harm from being repeated. Since people are generally reluctant to make formal complaints the numbers actually made are only a rough indication of satisfaction with NHS services. If formal complaints are to be a better indicator of levels of harm the NHS complaints procedures must be improved further. In particular the position with regard to complaints made in relation to the private sector requires urgent attention. People treated within the private sector do not have access to a substantial complaints procedure or the opportunity of support that was offered by CHCs to NHS users. Furthermore, it is possible that they carry a higher risk of being subject to harm (Ritchie Report, 2000). In the interests of the public, the tests and levels of accountability that the NHS and its staff are subject to should be extended to the private sector.

## Reducing harm in health care: lessons from the CHCs

In order to minimise harm in health care nurses and others working in health care should:

i. be familiar with the complaints procedures and relevant documentation
ii. support those who wish to complain by giving them clear information on the systems in place and the procedures required
iii. where appropriate, refer them on to individuals or bodies able to support them through the complaints procedures
iv. facilitate a culture of openness and communicate effectively with patients/clients and their significant others
v. use information gained from complaints to prevent errors and other forms of harm from being repeated
vi. lobby for the NHS complaints procedures to be open and accessible to complainants
vii. lobby for complaints procedures and quality assurance mechanisms, of the level used in the NHS, for the private sector.

# References

Anon (1991) GP: who watches the watchdogs? *Pulse*. 30 November, **46**, 16.

Association of Community Health Councils for England and Wales (1999) *Telemedicine*. Association of Community Health Councils for England and Wales, London.

Baker, R. (2001) *Harold Shipman's Clinical Practice 1974–1998*. Department of Health, London.

BBC News Online (2001) 'Wayne was in a lot of pain'. 19 April
http://news.bbc.co.uk/hi/english/health/newsid_1285000/128570.stm

Bristol Royal Infirmary Inquiry (2001) *Learning from Bristol. The report of the public inquiry into children's heart surgery at the Bristol Royal Infirmary, 1984–1995*. Department of Health, London.

Burke, A. (1997) *Hungry in Hospital?* Association of Community Health Councils for England and Wales, London.

Burke, A & Benham, M. (2001) *Nationwide Casualty Watch*. Association of Community Health Councils for England and Wales, London.

Chester, M. (2000) *'Fair Comment': How the threat of defamation undermines the NHS complaints system*. Association of Community Health Councils for England and Wales, London.

Commission on the NHS (2000) *New Life for Health*. Vintage, London.

Community Health Councils Regulations 1996 (SI 640). The Stationery Office, London.

Community Health Councils (Amendment) Regulations 2000 (SI 657) The Stationery Office, London.

Coulter, A. (2002) After Bristol: putting patients at the centre. *British Medical Journal*. **324**, 648–651.

Crompton, S. (2001) Patient rights under threat. *The Times*. 2 January, p. 8.

DoH (1999) *Supporting Doctors, Protecting Patients*. Department of Health, London.

DoH (2000a) *An Organisation with a Memory. Report of an expert group on learning from adverse events in the NHS chaired by the Chief Medical Officer*. The Stationery Office, London.

DoH (2000b) *Patients will benefit from private sector partnership*. Press statement 31 October, London.

DoH (2000c) *The NHS Plan: A plan for investment. A plan for reform*. Department of Health, London.

DoH (2001a) *Reforming the NHS Complaints Procedure: A listening document*. London.

DoH (2001b) *Handling Complaints: Monitoring the NHS complaints procedures. England. Financial Year 2000–01*.
http://www.doh.gov.uk/nhscomplaints/index.html

DoH (2001c) *Casualty Watch*. Department of Health statement, 28 March, London.

DoH (2001d) *Building a Safer NHS for Patients: Implementing 'An Organisation with a Memory'.* The Stationery Office, London.

DoH (2002) *Learning from Bristol: The Department of Health's response to the Report of the Public Inquiry into children's heart surgery at the Bristol Royal Infirmary 1984–1995.* The Stationery Office, London.

Ellis, N. (1996) *An Analysis of the Complaints Work of CHCs.* Association of Community Health Councils for England and Wales, London.

Griffith, B. (1997) *CHCs Making a Difference.* Association of Community Health Councils for England and Wales, London.

Health and Social Care Act 2001. The Stationery Office, London.

Healy, P. (1998) Role call. *Health Service Journal.* **108**, 13.

Hogg, C. (1996) *Back from the Margins. Which future for Community Health Councils?* Institute of Health Services Management, London.

Insight Management Consulting (1996) *Resourcing and Performance Management in Community Health Councils.* Final report. Department of Health, London.

Jain, A. & Ogden, J. (1999) General practitioners' experiences of patients' complaints: qualitative study. *British Medical Journal.* **318**, 1596–1599.

Kennedy, I., Howard, R., Jarman, B. & Maclean, M. (2000) *The Inquiry into the Management of Care of Children Receiving Complex Heart Surgery at the Bristol Royal Infirmary. Interim report – removal and retention of human material.* Bristol Royal Infirmary, Bristol.

National Health Service Act 1973. Her Majesty's Stationery Office, London.

National Health Service Act 1977. Her Majesty's Stationery Office, London.

National Health Service Reform and Health Care Professions Act 2002. The Stationery Office, London.

NMC (2002) *Code of Professional Conduct.* Nursing & Midwife Council, London.

Pollock, A. Rowland, D. & Vickers, N (2001) *Briefing note for the general election on health and privatisation.* 24 May. Health Policy and Health Services Research Unit, University College, London.

Public Interest Disclosure Act 1998. The Stationery Office, London.

Ritchie Report (2000) *Report of the Inquiry into Quality and Practice Within the National Health Service Arising from the Actions of Rodney Ledward.* Department of Health, London.

Robinson, J. (2001) *A Parent's View.* Statement by an Alder Hey parent. Personal communication from J. Robinson to the Association of Community Health Councils for England and Wales.

Royal College of Nursing (1996) *RCN statement on feeding and nutrition in hospitals.* RCN Press office to ACHCEW.

Royal College of Nursing (2000) *RCN General Secretary calls Casualty Watch findings 'A National Scandal'.* RCN press statement. 1 February, London.

Tameside and Glossop CHC (2001) *Tameside and Glossop Annual Report 2000/2001.* Tameside and Glossop CHC, Ashton-under-Lyne.

UKCC (1997) *UKCC says nurses have responsibility for the feeding of patients.*

United Kingdom Central Council for Nursing, Midwifery and Health Visiting press statement 8 May, London.

Wallace, H. & Mulcahy, L. (1999) *Cause for Complaint? An evaluation of the effectiveness of the NHS complaints procedure.* Public Law Project, London.

Williams, M. (1998) A Local Vision – results of the keeping care local feasibility study. Paper given at a Telemedicine Conference in Cardiff. Unpublished, Ceredigion CHC.

Wong, K. (1999) *1000 Years Experience in NHS Complaints. The evidence of Community Health Council Officers.* Barnet Community Health Council.

York Health Economics Consortium (2001) *NHS Complaints Procedure National Evaluation Report.* Department of Health, London.

# 9. Nurse Diagnosed Myocardial Infarction – Hidden Nurse Work and Iatrogenic Risk

*Denise Flisher and Marilyn Burn*

## Introduction

There have been considerable changes in the medical treatment and nursing care of patients with coronary heart disease since the early 1980s following the introduction of thrombolytic drugs for the treatment of acute myocardial infarction (AMI). These drugs have radically changed the management of such patients with their potential for re-perfusing ischaemic myocardium (improving the circulation to heart muscle) and thereby reducing mortality rates. In this chapter, we discuss how much added responsibility is placed on individual nurses by innovations such as nurse-led thrombolysis. This is explored in terms of the changing nature of modern practice and whether these new roles are desirable, beneficial for the patient, or wanted by the majority of coronary care nursing staff.

We will outline how an Acute Hospital Trust has attempted to reduce the time from admission to the accident and emergency (A&E) department, to administration of the thrombolytic drug, the so-called door-to-needle time. It could be argued that a coronary care nurse with the appropriate knowledge, training and experience has the ability to reduce this time. We will argue the case for nurse-led thrombolysis, discussing not only the benefits, but also the potential risk of harm to the patient that such a policy may engender. Finally it is noted how few studies have been carried out into the possible limitations and risks of thrombolysis.

## *Thrombolysis for acute myocardial infarction*

Heart disease remains a huge health problem in England and is a significant cause of death, killing over 110,000 people in 1998 including more than 41,000 under the age of 75. Furthermore, England has one of the highest death rates from heart disease in the world and the government has chosen it as a health priority (DoH, 2000). Thrombolysis is a process whereby a specific drug dissolves the clot without causing general anticoagulation in other systems. The plasminogen is converted to plasmin enabling it to dissolve the clot (Underhill *et al.*, 1990). A number of studies (GISSI, 1986; ISIS-2, 1988) have shown that this treatment appears to reduce mortality by 15% and saves 28 lives per 1000. The myocardial damage is restricted, potentially resulting in smaller infarctions and therefore fewer fatal outcomes. The benefit gained from administration of thrombolytic drugs is dependent on how soon after the onset of symptoms it is given (Julian, 1988). Pell *et al.* (1992) established that if the therapy is administered within six hours of the onset of symptoms there is a marked reduction in mortality. Others, like Ryan *et al.* (1997), argue that if the thrombolysis is given within two hours of occlusion there will be significant myocardial salvage – less heart muscle will be damaged. The drugs used in the thrombolysis programme referred to here are *streptokinase, tissue-type plasminogen activator* (TPA) and *reteplase*.

In England, the National Service Framework (NSF) for Coronary Heart Disease (DoH, 2000) attempted to set a clear national standard and identified a benchmark door-to-needle time of 20 minutes. In other words, once a person suffering from an acute AMI is admitted to hospital they should be assessed and thrombolysed, if this is the appropriate treatment, within 20 minutes. In order to achieve this 'gold standard', organisational changes have been required in the way patients are assessed and treated.

## *The nurse's role in thrombolysis*

As an acute and complex intervention, thrombolysis was originally undertaken by medical staff. More recently Quinn (1995) and Hood *et al.* (1998) offer clear support for nurse initiated thrombolysis, provided that the nurse in question works within the Code of Professional Conduct (NMC, 2002). Nurse-led thrombolysis was first tested by Quinn (1995) in a study to determine whether or not a nurse could safely assess a patient with regard to recognition of AMI and initiate appropriate thrombolysis. His findings showed that experienced coronary care nurses were able to assess patients as well as junior doctors. Similar findings were reported by Julian (1994) who demonstrated that experienced coronary care nurses' skills in electrocardiogram (ECG) interpretation appeared not only equal to, but in some cases better than, those of junior medical colleagues. In another study which examined ways of reducing door-to-needle times, Westwood and Prosser (1997) concluded that the use of critical care pathways, where the nurses and doctors combined their clinical notes, reduced paperwork and increased collaboration enhancing the prompt diagnosis of myocardial infarction. Somauroo *et al.* (1999) produced a study to determine whether or not a specialist nurse or nurses would improve the door-to-needle times. The authors concluded that with such an appointment their door-to-needle times had dramatically improved, with 100% of patients receiving thrombolysis within 60 minutes.

As already mentioned, large clinical trials have shown thrombolytic drugs to reduce mortality rates when administered to patients presenting with acute myocardial infarction (GISSI, 1986; ISIS-2, 1988). However, Julian (1988) suggested that although thrombolysis could save lives, it was dependent on the timeliness of its administration. When deciding how to introduce a so-called fast track system into our own hospital, using coronary care nurses to reduce door-to-needle times for patients presenting with AMI, many factors had to be taken into consideration and difficulties overcome. These included the levels of knowledge, skills and experience that the nurse would require and the impact of extending the role and responsibilities of the coronary care nurse in this sphere of practice. The innovation made some staff question whether this was how they wanted to take their vision of nursing forward, and how this extended role would be accepted by medical and nursing staff, both within coronary care unit (CCU) and the accident and emergency department.

Critical care environments are often perceived as one of the more 'glamorous' areas of the health service (Briggs, 1991), where nurses collaborate with medical staff and can enjoy greater mutual respect and autonomy than in ward environments. This in turn gives them greater confidence and willingness to take on the challenges and demands that role expansion makes on them. Personal experience certainly found this to be the case at this Hospital Trust amongst the majority of the CCU nurses when presented with the challenge of nurse-led thrombolysis. Concerns regarding possible errors in diagnosis and management, and the possibility of having to deal with any adverse consequences of thrombolysis in the unfamiliar work area of A&E, were voiced. This resulted in a core of four nurses initially participating in the administration of thrombolysis in A&E, but soon every CCU nurse assessed as competent was keen to join in. Benner *et al*. (1996, 2000) state that one of the nurse's major functions is to diagnose and monitor a patient's condition and to manage rapidly changing situations. Recognition for such skills is often not forthcoming, so this major area of nurses' actual practice is not legitimised and remains an example of the 'hidden' work that nurses do. Experienced CCU nursing staff are closely involved in the diagnosis of AMI and are heavily relied upon by junior medical staff. There is a risk that this work and therefore this expertise within nursing can remain hidden.

## The doctor–nurse relationship

In recent years, traditional boundaries between differing health care professionals have come under scrutiny, with authors such as Beardshaw and Robinson (1990) arguing the need for a fundamental shift in roles and attitudes in order to address the poor esteem and high nurse wastage within the National Health Service. Relationships between doctors and nurses have historically had a rigid hierarchical structure linked to the cultural ethos of the British class system. MacKay (1993) observes that nurses trained abroad may not exhibit such constraints and consequently can enjoy a more equal relationship with the medical profession, having little perception of any disparity between themselves and doctors. An area of potential conflict with regard to who is best based placed to diagnose and initiate thrombolysis is the occupational boundary between medical and nursing staff. Traditionally the doctor has maintained a dominant role, with the nurse implementing care which the doctor has prescribed (Watson, 1999), but these roles need to be challenged, and more importantly changed if nurse-led thrombolysis is to be successful.

For many years, nurses themselves have perpetuated these beliefs, perhaps content with the public's stereotypical view of them as 'angels', unwilling or unable to work together and demand recognition for their contribution to health care. The Department of Health White Paper on reform of the NHS signalled the belief that skills and roles across all professions in the NHS needed to be reviewed stating:

'There have been many developments in recent years in the better use of nursing staff, but the Government believes that there is still

174

scope for more progress at local level... Local managers, in consultation with their professional colleagues, will be expected to re-examine all areas of work to identify the most cost-effective use of professional skills. This may involve a re-appraisal of traditional patterns and practices. Examples include the extended role of nurses to cover specific duties normally undertaken by junior doctors in areas of high technology care and in casualty departments.'

DoH, 1989 p. 15

There are then pressures to encourage nurses, such as those involved in the care and treatment of people with AMI, to expand their practice and take on new roles.

It could be argued that in a Health Service with limited resources this is an attempt to reduce costs, as it is far cheaper to employ a nurse than it is a doctor. It is clear that the traditional, subservient nursing role is changing with the introduction of developments such as primary nursing, nursing development units, the scope of professional practice and increasing opportunities for clinical practice development posts (Kendrick, 1995). Holmes (1991 p. 16) argued:

'Clinical leaders will create an environment in which therapeutic relationships with patients and collaborative relationships with other health care professionals are possible. Effective application of the skills of leadership, therefore, expands the role of nurses, setting a standard for professional practice and helping to guide its development. This can only be of benefit both to patients and to the quality of the care they receive.'

There needs to be, therefore, a close and effective working relationship between nursing and medical staff but changes to occupational roles can be difficult to implement.

Clinical autonomy and self-regulation are guiding principles of the medical profession, and Johnson & Boss (1991) maintain that as medical work is highly personal and closely involved with matters of life and death, it has traditionally been given high levels of autonomy. Interventions, which seek to change clinical practice, especially in acute health care environments, impinge on this autonomy and disturb the clinician's sense of security, thus potentially creating resistance to change. In addition, qualities seen as attractive and positive in men, and medicine has been an occupation dominated by men, may be viewed very differently if

175

exhibited by a woman, who may be seen as sacrificing her femininity should she display the characteristics of assertiveness, decisiveness, authority and power.

Such gender divisions have classically been exhibited in the 'doctor–nurse' game as described by Stein (1967; Stein *et al.*, 1990). This is a performance played out between doctor and nurse whereby a knowledgeable and experienced nurse feigns inequality to a doctor. Nurses disguise their skills by feeding the doctor with information and advice, ensuring that the doctor appears in a favourable light, appears to make the crucial decisions, and does not lose face in front of the patient. This helps to maintain the patient's confidence in the doctor's ability, and reduces the number of errors made. Nurses can defend such a position by stating that these games help maintain good working relationships with medical staff. However, in reality the patient becomes a pawn in this game, being a passive onlooker, frequently unaware of the tensions that can remain in the traditional patriarchal doctor–nurse relationship (Sweet & Norman, 1995). This game, according to Sweet and Norman in a review of the literature on the subject, inhibits communication and probably, therefore, contributes to the occurrence of adverse health care events even after the reduction of errors through the nurses' hidden work is taken into consideration.

## Expanding the role of the nurse

In arguing for a leading role by nurses these issues were considered and a clear case put for challenging such notions and allowing nurses to take on a fuller role in thrombolysis. Patients admitted directly to A&E have the potential of a much faster door-to-needle time, and the nursing staff of the CCU were determined to make nurse-led thrombolysis work, believing it would improve patient care and could possibly save lives. We cited our accountability for care and the fundamental requirement to promote and safeguard the interests of individual patients/clients as laid down in the Code of Professional Conduct (NMC, 2002).

In order for nurse-led thrombolysis to be a success, much thought and preparation was required prior to proceeding with the initiative. Only experienced, skilled, competent and confident nurses were permitted to take on the thrombolysis role. The success of nurse-led thrombolysis would depend on effective collaboration with, and cooperation from, both the doctors and nurses of A&E. We understood their concerns and it was agreed that the doctors in A&E would always be consulted and the ECGs discussed whenever a patient was seen, and reassurance was given that they would be fully involved when a patient was thrombolysed. This has allowed the current system to be implemented – working in a collaborative team, coordinating the work of two acute areas, coronary care and A&E.

Although there is a growing desire in some nurses for greater autonomy and a wish to pursue a wider range of extended or specialist roles, there are those who fear that this will lead to the caring aspects of the role being devalued and passed on to unqualified support staff. Some fear that the technical skills gained will be at the expense of the interpersonal skills and qualities which have been the central element of a nurse's role – that the nature of nursing will change and many traditional nursing duties will be lost in the rush to acquire skills which have historically been associated with medicine rather than nursing. This is discussed in the work of Watson (1999), who believes that nurses are moving beyond the high-tech, 'cure at all cost' ethos of our time. Watson goes on to say that nurses need to rediscover the caring art and put it back into their nursing practice, that western medicine has the ethos of 'cure at all costs', where very few are 'allowed' simply to die in hospital and be afforded good quality nursing care without the use of modern machines and interventions. However, this creates a tension for those nurses wishing to participate in thrombolysis in the sense that the nurse is asked to bridge the care–cure boundary that is commonly associated with nursing and medicine respectively (Dunlop, 1986). This dichotomy, the simplistic separation of care from cure is widely accepted by the public but does not reflect the potentially therapeutic nature of the nurse–patient relationship (Watson, 1998). These arguments do not mean that the nurse should not be initiating thrombolysis but that a way forward needs to be found to facilitate nurse-led thrombolysis without compromising other less technological aspects of the role. Using Watson's (1999) and Benner *et al.*'s (2000) work it is also possible to suggest that nurses are well placed to help make decisions about the need for and appropriateness of thrombolytic therapy due to their intimate understanding of the patient's predicament.

The senior medical staff at this particular Hospital Trust were at first reluctant to accept that the success of nurse-initiated thrombolysis would be dependent on the CCU nurses' ability to recognise those patients who required the service. They were prepared to allow the nurses to assess only those patients admitted via GPs, but not those admitted directly to A&E. Their argument was that it was not the role of a nurse to make a diagnosis, and that the senior house officers (SHOs) would miss the experience of reading ECGs. This reluctance may in some part be explained by the protection of territorial boundaries (Hugman, 1991), and disagreements when members of one discipline exploit a hierarchical relationship with other members of the interdisciplinary team. Hoekelman (1994) believes that collaboration between medicine and nursing is hampered by a basic dishonesty in nurse–physician interactions, with sexism, educational differences, economic discrepancies, classism and misunderstanding of each other's roles all being identified as root causes. However, the initial reservations were overcome and consent obtained from the relevant medical staff and nurse-led thrombolysis initiated.

## Is thrombolysis just another task?

There is a risk that the delegation of key aspects of the diagnosis and administration of thrombolysis to nurses could be perceived as simply the authorising of a new task. As Ackroyd (1993) observes, all grades of nurses often express high levels of job satisfaction, employing skills to decide on the order and priority of tasks together with hard physical effort. In other words, not all tasks are uninteresting, and some are deceptively complex. Walsh (2000) argues that the greatest criticism of the extended role of the nurse is that it can be seen as having been reduced to a series of tasks. It could be argued that if nursing is drifting back towards task orientation, there could be a danger of budget-focused managers training specific groups, perhaps technicians with National Vocational Qualifications (NVQ) level 2 or 3, to carry out such tasks in place of a more expensive qualified nurse. It could be envisaged, therefore, that technicians might be asked to undertake thrombolysis. It is suggested here that this might be an inappropriate step and the reasons for this assertion are discussed below.

Mitchell (1997) has suggested that nurses administer quality care, although it is acknowledged here that nursing has itself been accused of a task-focused approach to care (for example Walsh & Ford, 1990) whereas technicians may tend not to develop rapport between themselves and the patient, resulting in task focusing and less effective communication. Mitchell also argues that a nurse has to make a clinical judgement about what to do next, for example, if the patient's blood pressure drops following thrombolysis, the nurse, through experience will instinctively know what to do. Similarly, Walsh (2000) notes that to complete a procedure successfully, a nurse needs to be able to respond effectively to unusual and unforeseen events that may occur during the procedure. Indeed, an appropriate response, what Benner *et al.* (2000) referred to as thinking-in-action in nursing practice, can be more important than the skills required in simply completing the task. Furthermore, Hansten and Washburn (1998) argue that clinical areas which have a higher proportion of registered nurses offer better quality care than those wards with a lower skill mix. This results in a better 'journey' for the patient as the first and last person the patient meets is usually the nurse.

Here, in the context of this complex aspect of clinical practice, it is argued that registered nurses are better placed to react to a range of situations whereas technicians and health care assistants may have a more limited range of responses and may require help and supervision from others. Nurses may also have strengths in relation to thrombolysis over and above those offered by junior, and perhaps even senior medical staff due to the range and quality of nurse–patient contact that they achieve (Birkhead, 1992; Julian, 1994).

## Experience and the advanced practitioner

There continues to be confusion regarding the various terms used to describe the nurse equipped to carry out a task as responsible as thrombolysis. The terms 'advanced nurse practitioner' and 'specialist practitioner' continue to confuse many, although it could be argued that the holding of an advanced practice award could indicate a specialist practitioner, a notion supported within the position statement of the UKCC (1996). The UKCC felt it was necessary for all specialist nurses to have been granted a post-registration qualification in a specific field. However, the employer must be satisfied through agreed criteria and protocols that such an award is accompanied by the appropriate level of skill, knowledge and experience. In many coronary care units in the UK these criteria might apply to a significant number of their nurses, and it should therefore be possible for them to utilise their skills in nurse-led thrombolysis, rather than leaving it to just one or two specialist practitioners. The Nursing and Midwifery Council (NMC, 2002) recently integrated the concept of the Scope of Practice into the *Professional Code of Conduct*.

Benner *et al.* (1996) describe experience as being a requisite for expertise, and the problem solving of a proficient or expert nurse can be attributed to the 'know-how' that is acquired through this experience. This is an important point as experience can build a powerful base upon which to make decisions such as those required in diagnosing a myocardial infarction and is also true of the decision process in thrombolysis. The appropriateness of the latter is of course dependent upon an accurate diagnosis. A nurse can be taught how to comprehensively assess a person suspected of developing or having had an AMI, and to recognise the relevant changes on an ECG and how to administer an appropriate thrombolytic drug. However, there are times when people present with atypical symptoms and the ECG may be difficult to interpret or the occurrence of a 'non-conventional' complication might occur following drug administration. Examples such as a thrombolytic rash, which may appear all over the body, or excruciating back pain seldom occur, but when they do happen it can be very frightening to both patient and practitioner. These complications are more likely to be seen by the experienced nurse and are not well described in the literature.

The framework offered by Burnard (1991) can help to structure the benefits that nurses can bring to thrombolysis and the limitations that they face in comparison with medical staff. Burnard identified three types of knowledge as being relevant to health care practice: *propositional*, *experiential* and *practical* (skills). Propositional knowledge includes theories and models, research and other literature – for want of a better expression, the theory behind it. Experiential knowledge is that gained from and through experience, and practical refers to the psychomotor tasks that we face. For convenience, as this later category is about skills, we shall use the term 'skills'.

Figure 9.1 shows these three types of knowledge and creates a crude model of how they can be applied to thrombolysis and the strengths that nursing and medical staff can have in relation to this. A plus sign (+) is used to represent the amount of knowledge held, with one plus equalling entry level knowledge, and three a significant amount of relevant knowledge, that held by an expert.

In terms of skills, both nursing and medical staff start with limited skills but have the potential to develop these fully. Such skills include the handling of equipment, including relevant monitors and ECG machines, and the drug administration process itself. Inexperienced medical staff will have a higher level of propositional knowledge than experienced nursing staff simply because of their preparation for the role and it is unlikely that even experienced nursing staff would be able to reach the same levels of propositional knowledge as a medical specialist. However, nursing staff can gain more experiential knowledge than medical staff because of the

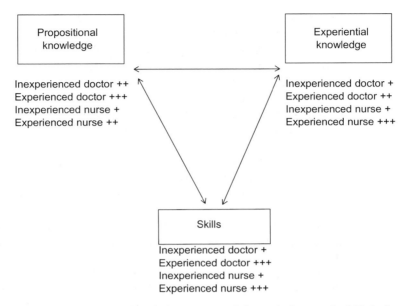

**Fig. 9.1** A comparison of the projected knowledge and skill balance between nursing and medical staff.

quality and quantity of contact that they will have with these patients. This includes experience gained from the admission and assessment process, through treatment and the subsequent care process. The continuity of this care ensures that nursing staff can gain an experiential advantage over medical staff.

Although Fig. 9.1 is a rather crude representation of a complex range of issues, it does help to illustrate some of the tensions discussed in this chapter. Although nurses may invariably have a propositional knowledge deficit in comparison with experienced medical staff, they have a richer experiential knowledge base to call upon to help them make judgements in acute clinical situations (Benner *et al.*, 2000). The time constraints that are part of the assessment and treatment process in thrombolysis mean that such insights can prove invaluable in making rapid, informed and accurate decisions.

The possibility of technicians undertaking thrombolysis could have associated risks using the framework offered in Fig. 9.1. They are likely to have a propositional knowledge deficit in comparison with the experienced nurse or doctor. Furthermore, and as asserted here in relation to medical staff, they are unlikely to build up the rich base of experiential knowledge seen in the experienced CCU nurse.

## *Reasons for delay in thrombolysis*

Having explored differences in knowledge base we return now to the practical issue of time delay. There have been a number of studies carried out that discuss the reasons for delay in initiating thrombolytic therapy.

The literature suggests that there are three significant causes of delay. The first presented by Birkhead (1992) and Herriot (1993) is delay by the patient in calling for help. Birkhead established that one of the major factors was the time that it took patients to present themselves to their own GP or to the local accident and emergency department and noted that patients with additional symptoms were more likely to call the emergency services and so arrive at the hospital sooner. Pell *et al.* (1992) argued in their study that most patients presented to hospital within three hours of the onset of their symptoms. He found that 50% of GP referrals to A&E were seen within 15 minutes of arrival at the hospital. However, Pell *et al.* did add that GPs recognised that those patients who self-referred to the casualty department had more severe symptoms and would therefore seek help at a faster rate.

The second cause of delay is pre-hospital examination and evaluation by the GP or ambulance crew, either of whom may find it difficult to establish intravenous access in the shocked patient if the procedure is attempted. Rawles (1997) suggested that some GPs carried out a full medical examination, called the ambulance for admission and when the crew arrived continued with another detailed assessment of the patient. This all added to the delay in arriving at hospital and the administration of thrombolysis.

The third delay occurs within the hospital where decisions as to whether or not the patient should receive thrombolysis would be taken. Some hospitals have initiated thrombolysis in the accident department, some on the coronary care unit and some on the acute admissions ward. Throughout the literature (Cobbe, 1994; McCabe & West, 1998; Flisher, 2000) there is overwhelming evidence to suggest that the third causal delay could be resolved by developing a streamlined procedure to facilitate early thrombolysis.

Flisher (1995) has suggested that the hospital delay from patient admission to the accident and emergency department to the administration of thrombolysis (door-to-needle time) was the result of system failure. The system adapted at this particular district hospital was one whereby the casualty officer examined the patient and made a provisional diagnosis of AMI. This patient was then referred to the admitting 'on-call' medical team who reconfirmed the diagnosis, admitted the patient to coronary care where there was a third examination by the registrar on call. It was at this point that thrombolytic therapy was administered. Flisher (1995) developed a new system which reduced the door-to-needle time from over 90 minutes to 30 minutes or less. This was achieved by an appropriately trained coronary care nurse going to the accident and emergency department, recording the ECG, making a diagnosis (which is confirmed by a doctor on CCU) and transferring the patient directly to the CCU. There the on-call registrar or SHO confirmed the diagnosis, completed the contra-indication checklist with the nurse and administered the appropriate thrombolytic drug. This procedure was termed 'fast track'.

Further progress has been made in establishing a faster door-to-needle time (Flisher, 2000). The 30-minute barrier could not be improved upon because of uncontrolled delays, such as waiting for analgesia before transfer to the coronary care unit, intravenous cannulation or waiting for porters. Therefore, the CCU nurse goes to the A&E department and records the ECG, he/she and the casualty officer then collaborate to make a diagnosis from the patient assessment and ECG. Together the assessment sheet is completed (Fig. 9.2), the appropriate drug is chosen as per protocol, and the therapy is given by the coronary care nurse in the A&E department. The drug is prescribed by the casualty doctor. Whilst the nurse has an expert understanding of patient assessment in this situation and of ECG reading, a reliable medical opinion remains important in taking the decision whether or not to initiate thrombolysis. The protocols and assessment sheet are reviewed on a yearly basis by the cardiology team and nurses on the CCU to ensure that any recent research is incorporated within these guidelines.

The nurse is trained to expect the unexpected in terms of complications and how to react accordingly. Knowledge in relation to the local drug policy is required, along with the drugs utilised within the role – aspirin, the actual thrombolytic itself and heparin. These are researched thoroughly before the extended role is assumed. The resulting door-to-needle time currently stands at 15 minutes or less and is termed 'accelerated fast track'. This is an example of excellent communication, collaboration by the different departments and a multidisciplinary approach to facilitate a faster door-to-needle time. But what risks might this procedure carry for patients and those staff charged with giving thrombolysis?

**MYOCARDIAL INFARCTION PATIENT ASSESSMENT FORM**

| *Patient addressograph (including NHS number)* | Q1 Amb.Incident no: ⬚⬚⬚⬚⬚⬚ | Q2 Ethnic origin: |
|---|---|---|
| | **Presentation:** | Q3 Admission diagnosis: |
| | Q4 Whom did patient call for help? | |

**Q5**
AFT: ☐     FT: ☐     Other: _____

| **Delays to treatment:** | Q6 Was reperfusion attempted? Yes ☐  ☐ No |
|---|---|

**Q7**

| | D D / M M / Y Y   H H : M M | **Therapy:** |
|---|---|---|
| Onset of symptoms: | ⬚⬚ / ⬚⬚ / ⬚⬚   ⬚⬚ : ⬚⬚ | Q8 ECG changes: |
| Call for help: | ⬚⬚ / ⬚⬚ / ⬚⬚   ⬚⬚ : ⬚⬚ | Q9 Where was treatment given? |
| Arrival of 1st responder: | ⬚⬚ / ⬚⬚ / ⬚⬚   ⬚⬚ : ⬚⬚ | Q10 Enzymes elevated >x2? Yes ☐  ☐ No |
| Arrival of Ambulance: | ⬚⬚ / ⬚⬚ / ⬚⬚   ⬚⬚ : ⬚⬚ | Diuretic treatment given? Yes ☐  ☐ No |
| Arrival at Hospital: | ⬚⬚ / ⬚⬚ / ⬚⬚   ⬚⬚ : ⬚⬚ | Peak CK: ⬚⬚⬚⬚ |
| Reperfusion treatment: | ⬚⬚ / ⬚⬚ / ⬚⬚   ⬚⬚ : ⬚⬚ | Troponin T result (if done): |

| Q12 Who initiated treatment? | Q11 Reason reperfusion treatment not given: |
|---|---|
| Q13 When and where was Aspirin given? | Q14 Was there a justified delay? Yes ☐  ☐ No |
| | Describe: |
| | Or other? |

| **Patient details and hospital course:** | Q15 Admission ward: | Q16 Admitting Consultant: |
|---|---|---|

**Q17 Previous medical history:**

| None ☐ | Previous AMI ☐ | Peripheral vascular disease ☐ | Cholesterol: |
|---|---|---|---|
| Treated diabetes ☐ | Treated hyperlipidaemia ☐ | Asthma ☐ | |
| Current smoker ☐ | Treated angina ☐ | Treated BP ☐ | ⬚⬚ • ⬚ mmol/L |

Final diagnosis:

Cause of death in hospital:

Date of death: ⬚⬚ / ⬚⬚ / ⬚⬚     Discharge date: ⬚⬚ / ⬚⬚ / ⬚⬚

| Secondary prevention: | | |
|---|---|---|
| Q18 B blocker: ☐   Aspirin: ☐ | ACE 1/AT2 blocker: ☐   Rehabilitation | Statin: ☐ |

| Treatment/investigations performed during admission or planned: |
|---|

| Q19 Exercise test: ☐   Coronary angio: ☐ | Echocardiograph: ☐   Coronary intervention: ☐ | Perfusion scanning: ☐ |
|---|---|---|

**Cardiac arrest:**

Q20 Date and time of 1st arrest    D D / M M / Y Y    H H : M M

Where did it occur? _____

Presenting rhythm: _____    Outcome: _____

Comments: _____

**Q21 *For CCU Use:***

Admitting Diagnosis: _____    Suggested by: _____

Indication for Thrombolysis:

| | Yes | No |
|---|---|---|
| Symptoms suggestive of MI: | | |
| Crushing chest pain for 15 mins – not relieved by rest, oxygen or GTN | Yes ☐ | No |
| Pain started within last 12 hours or within 24 hours if ongoing pain | Yes ☐ | No |

12 lead ECG shows:

| | Yes | No |
|---|---|---|
| ST segment elevation of at least 1 mm in two of limb leads | Yes ☐ | No |
| and/or ST segment elevation of at least 2 mm in two of the chest leads | Yes ☐ | No |
| Left Bundle Branch Block not known to be old | Yes ☐ | No |

Contra-indications for Accelerated or fast track Thrombolysis:    (Present or Suspected)

| -previous CVA (within last 12 months) | Yes ☐ ☐ No | -active peptic ulceration | Yes ☐ ☐ No |
|---|---|---|---|
| -recent streptococcal infection (known) | Yes ☐ ☐ No | -known allergy to the drug (or had before in the last year) | Yes ☐ ☐ No |
| -resent surgery (up to 6 days) | Yes ☐ ☐ No | -possible aortic dissection back pain, unequal blood pressures | Yes ☐ ☐ No |
| -prolonged & traumatic chest compressions | Yes ☐ ☐ No | -possible pregnancy | Yes ☐ ☐ No |
| -anticoagulation therapy (obtain INR) | Yes ☐ ☐ No | -recently inserted central or arterial line | Yes ☐ ☐ No |
| -diastolic blood pressure above 120mmHg -systolic blood pressure above 200mmHg | BP = ☐☐☐ · ☐☐ | | Yes ☐ ☐ No |

**Age and diabetes (retinopathy) are no longer contra-indications**
**FEW OF THESE CONTRA-INDICATIONS ARE ABSOLUTE - SEEK SHO ADVICE**

Clear indications for thrombolysis?    Yes ☐  ☐ No    Verbal consent obtained? ☐

If yes, Thrombolytic agent chosen:    Rapilysin ☐    Streptokinase ☐

Signature of Nurse for admin of thrombolysis: _____    Printed name: _____    Date: D D / M M / Y Y

Signature of Nurse completing form: _____    Printed name: _____    Date: D D / M M / Y Y

**Fig. 9.2**   Myocardial infarction patient assessment form.

## *Early thrombolysis: the iatrogenic risk*

### Timeframe and error

The concept of an accelerated fast track system for patients presenting with acute myocardial infarction, with its emphasis on delivery of thrombolysis within a very short timeframe, increases the potential for doing the patient harm. As demonstrated in the Introduction and Chapter 2 of this book, error rates are known to be high in health care (Brennan *et al.*, 1991; Leape, 1991; Wilson *et al.*, 1995; Vincent *et al.*, 2001) and there is little reason to suppose that this will be any different in the diagnosis and treatment of AMI. As the nurse and medical staff strive to initiate thrombolysis within the 20 minute window, as suggested in the NSF (DoH, 2000), they may be tempted to rush the assessment, which includes the identification of any contraindications to the drugs used, resulting in potentially life threatening consequences. The need for thoroughness has to be balanced against the drive for a shorter door-to-needle time maximising the amount of heart muscle saved. Rawles (1997) suggests that those patients requiring thrombolytic therapy should be afforded the same urgency as those suffering a cardiac arrest, in other words, they must be treated immediately. However, apart from the difficulty inherent in making a full assessment and accurate diagnosis, including the identification of any other significant health problems, complications can arise from the side effects of this particular drug therapy. These range, for example, from bleeding gums to extensive cerebral bleeds resulting in debilitating and potentially fatal cerebral vascular accidents (strokes).

These pressures are real and beyond the control, in terms of the demand for such treatment, of the local clinicians. In the UK the National Service Framework for Coronary Heart Disease (DoH, 2000) seeks to reduce not only the door-to-needle time to 20 minutes, but also to reduce the call-to-needle time to 60 minutes or less. The call-to-needle time reflects the time from when the patient calls for help (e.g. from the GP or the emergency services on the telephone) to the administration of thrombolysis. The underpinning theme is to reduce these times, but this may be to the detriment of the patient if the possibility of error and other adverse events is not taken into consideration.

### Transfer

Although cannulated and given pain relief in A&E, a patient who is transferred in the acute stages of AMI having just received thrombolysis, along corridors and in a lift to the CCU, also has the potential to suffer harm. The risk of life threatening arrhythmias during the transfer process will always be present, necessitating the initiation of cardio-pulmonary resuscitation in an unsuitable and uncontrolled environment. Such transfers are inevitable where the admissions department is separate from the coronary care unit and the pressures of door-to-needle times have to be met. However, in the seven years the authors have been involved in fast tracking patients with an acute myocardial infarction, not one has required resuscitation during transfer. This illustrates the nurses' abilities to assess the patient thoroughly and recognise whether a patient is stable enough for transfer.

## Limitations of thrombolytic therapy

In addition to the increase in risk inherent in time limited interventions, there is some evidence to suggest that there are limitations in the effectiveness of thrombolysis beyond the risks of haemorrhage and adverse drug reactions. Chareonthaitawee *et al.* (2000) argue that although there is overwhelming evidence to suggest that the earlier the thrombolysis is undertaken the greater the myocardial salvage, there will also be more reperfused myocardium prone to re-infarction. They argue that early thrombolysis increases the likelihood of re-infarction within six weeks because the viable myocardium preserved by the thrombolysis is susceptible to further episodes of ischaemia and infarction. The overall results of this study involving 2770 patients concluded that the beneficial effect of thrombolysis was maximised if given within two hours of the onset of symptoms. However, although re-infarction rates were higher in this group, as previously discussed, the overall mortality rates were much less. In this study it was found that patients having recovered initially from their AMI, were still faced with more rehabilitation, larger infarctions and slower recovery after infarction.

Limitations in the use of thrombolysis in the elderly population have also been identified. Thiemann *et al.* (2000) carried out a large retrospective study of 2673 patients between 76 and 86 years old who received intravenous thrombolytic therapy for AMI. The study, which included comparisons with a slightly younger group (65 to 75 years old) concluded that thrombolytic therapy for those over 75 years old was unlikely to confer survival benefits and might carry a significant survival disadvantage. The survival advantages for the younger group were said to be consistent with randomised trials of the therapy. Commenting on Thiemann *et al.*'s work, De Silvey (2000) highlighted the complexities faced by those making decisions with regard to the initiation of such treatment in the elderly population. It is noted that assessment is crucial in determining which individuals are likely to benefit from this therapy. Such assessment may prove more time consuming with the elderly due to the sensory deficits and more complex health histories that commonly go with the ageing process.

## Moving to a 20 minute door-to-needle time

Time, however, is at a premium in thrombolytic therapy. The NSF (DoH, 2000) clearly indicates that the door-to-needle times should be further reduced to 20 minutes or less by April 2003 and this time is counted from the moment when the ambulance stops at the hospital. By the time the patient is wheeled into the appropriate area, be it A&E or the CCU, undressed (sometimes removing several layers of clothing), an ECG recorded, interpreted and an assessment completed including contraindications to thrombolysis, 20 minutes may have already elapsed. In a system increasingly driven by comparisons between Acute Hospital Trusts on goal performance, such as door-to-needle times, pressures will increase on clinical staff to meet such goals and safety may possibly be compromised.

## Consent

It must also be questioned, in our quest for rapid door-to-needle times, whether the major side effects of the drug therapy are ever fully explained to the patient? The patient with AMI suffers a potentially life threatening condition, one that is clearly understood by the public as such, and will be asked to make decisions with regard to treatment often under the influence of potent analgesia, for example diamorphine. In this scenario the patients rely on clinicians to render their condition stable, and will be likely to agree, under such pressure, to almost any form of treatment. Consent is obtained for thrombolysis by word of mouth or by written consent depending on local policy. However, with a time restricted treatment the side effects and pitfalls of thrombolysis may not always be fully explained to the patient. Emphasis on the risk of bleeding is often played down, and the major complications may rarely or seldom be mentioned, namely debilitating stroke.

The danger in terms of obtaining consent, is the temptation to cut corners and it is important that protocols are strictly followed, even if it means a delay in commencing thrombolysis. There is even the potential to forget to complete the contraindication list. The Department of Health, in its guidance on consent for treatment and examination (DoH, 2001), make it clear that the consultant remains responsible for the overall quality of care the patient receives, but the task of gaining consent for specific treatments or investigations can be delegated to other clinicians. These clinicians must have sufficient knowledge relevant to the procedure and understand the risks involved. As De Silvey (2000) concludes, thrombolytic therapy for AMI should be administered with caution and a thorough understanding of the risk/benefits involved. To meet the requirements of informed consent, these risks also need to be explained to the patient.

## Conclusion

There is good evidence to suggest that early thrombolysis can save lives and enhance the quality of life of those that survive acute myocardial infarction. The optimum time at which to begin the administration of the therapy remains a point of contention in the medical literature, but in the UK clear goals have been set through the National Service Framework for Coronary Heart Disease (DoH, 2000). The questions of who administers the drug and where have created debate amongst medical and nursing staff, challenging the historical boundaries of responsibility between the two occupational groups. This has resulted in an emerging consensus of opinion that nurses can gain the necessary experience and skills to administer a potentially harmful drug in the form of thrombolytic therapy safely in cooperation with suitably experienced medical staff. In terms of the propositional knowledge base nurses operate from, it is argued here that it is unlikely that this will be as strong as that of medical staff, but the quality of experiential knowledge gained by nurses can, to some extent, compensate for this. This experiential advantage is derived from nurse's close contact with a wide range of patients suffering from AMI and the continuity inherent in the nurse–patient relationship. Medical staff will find it difficult to gain such an experiential foundation due to the more transient nature of patient contact that their role involves.

Discussion on the potential harm to patients from this drug therapy has also been briefly described. The studies by Chareonthaitawee *et al.* (2000) and Thiemann *et al.* (2000) are examples of the complexity of this intervention and its possible limitations. Those involved in this treatment process will need to be familiar with the relevant ongoing research especially as the effect of reducing the door-to-needle time to 20 minutes is likely, on the evidence cited here, to increase the risk of errors being made and impact upon the process of gaining consent. This time limit may also increase the chance of patients being wrongly treated for an AMI when they have another health problem. Thrombolysis is an acute, expensive, technological intervention that can have a positive effect on the health of many of those suffering an acute myocardial infarction. It is also a potentially dangerous intervention that requires accurate and comprehensive patient assessment and close cooperation between members of the multidisciplinary team. Nursing and medical staff need to work together to combine the knowledge, skills and experience that they bring to clinical practice in a way that benefits those patients that might require thrombolytic therapy.

## Reducing harm in nurse-led thrombolysis

In order to minimise unnecessary harm in nurse-led thrombolysis the nurse should:

i.   not accept the role unless adequately prepared in terms of relevant theoretical knowledge, experience and skills

ii.  endeavour to work honestly and effectively with medical staff during the diagnostic process and work within local policies and procedures

iii. communicate concerns regarding the suitability of patients for treatment to fellow staff

iv.  ensure that effective support systems are in place for nurses undertaking thrombolysis and that roles are defined within and between the different departments involved

v.   keep abreast of the changing research in this area and remain sensitive to the implications of this to practice

vi.  encourage effective case evaluation between the various health care staff involved, especially when patients present or respond to treatment in unusual ways

vii. ensure that research undertaken in relation to thrombolysis reflects the complexity of practice through the honest reporting of adverse events and complications.

# *References*

Ackroyd, S. (1993) Nurses, management and morale: a diagnosis of decline in the NHS hospital service. In: *Interprofessional Relations in Health Care* (eds K. Soothill, L. Mackay & C. Webb), pp. 222–239. Edward Arnold, London.

Beardshaw, W. & Robinson, R. (1990) *New for Old: Prospects for nursing in the 1990s.* King's Fund, London.

Benner, P., Tanner, C. & Chesla, C. (1996) *Expertise in Nursing Practice.* Springer Publishing Company, New York.

Benner, P., Hooper-Kyriakidis, P. & Stannard, D. (2000) *Clinical Wisdom and Interventions in Critical Care. A thinking-in-action approach*. W. B. Saunders Company, Philadelphia.

Birkhead, J. S. (1992) Time delays in provision of thrombolytic treatment in six district hospitals. *British Medical Journal*. **305**, 445–448.

Boreham, N.C., Shea, C. E. & Mackway-Jones K. (2000) Clinical risk in the hospital emergency department in the UK. *Social Science and Medicine*. **51**, 83–91.

Brennan, T. A., Leape, L. L., Laird, N. M., Hebert, L., Localio, A. R., Lawthers, A. G., Newhouse, J. P., Weiler, P. C. & Hiatt, H. H. (1991) Incidence of adverse events and negligence in hospitalized patients. Results of the Harvard Medical Practice Study I. *New England Journal of Medicine*. **324**, 370–376.

Briggs, D. (1991) Critical care nurse's role – traditional or expanded/extended. *Intensive Care Nursing* 7, 223–229.

Burnard, P. (1991) *Learning Human Skills*, 2nd edition. Butterworth Heinemann, London.

Chareonthaitawee, P., Gibbons, R. J., Roberts, R. S., Christian, T. F., Burns, R. & Yusef, S. (2000) The impact of time to thrombolytic treatment on outcome in patients with acute myocardial infarction. *Heart*. **84**, 142–148.

Cobbe, S. (1994) Thrombolysis in myocardial infarction. *British Medical Journal*. **308**, 216–217.

DoH (1989) *Working for Patients*. HMSO, London.

DoH (2000) *National Service Framework for Coronary Heart Disease. Modern Standard and Service Models*. Department of Health, London.

DoH (2001) *Reference Guide to Consent for Examination or Treatment*. Department of Health, London.

De Silvey, D. L. (2000) Risk of thrombolysis in the elderly. *American Journal of Geriatric Cardiology*. **9**, 292–293.

Dunlop, M. J. (1986) Is a science of caring possible? *Journal of Advanced Nursing*. **11**, 661–670.

Flisher, D. C. (1995) Fast track: early thrombolysis. *British Journal of Nursing*. **4**, 562–565.

Flisher, D. C. (2000) Fast track: early thrombolysis In: *Aspects of Cardiovascular Nursing* (eds J. Cruickshank, M. Bradbury & S. Ashurst), pp. 98–102. Quay Books and Mark Allen Publishing, Dinton, Wilts.

GISSI (Gruppo Italiano per lo Studio della Streptochinaisi nell' Infarto Miocardio) (1986) Long term effects of intravenous thrombolysis in acute myocardial infarction: final reports of the GISSI study. *The Lancet*. **2**, 871–874.

Hansten, R. J. & Washburn, M. J. (1998) *Clinical Delegation Skills: A handbook for professional practice*, 2nd edn. Gaithersburg, Aspen, CO.

Herriot, A. G., Brecker, S. J. & Coltart, D. J. (1993) Delay in the presentation after myocardial infarction. *Journal of the Royal Society of Medicine*. **86**, 642–644.

Hoekelman, R. A. (1994) Nurse–physician relationships; problems and solutions. Rush-Presbyterian-St. Luke's Medical Centre, Chicago. Unpublished paper.

Holmes, S. (1991) Clinical leadership: a role for the advanced practitioner? *Journal of Advances in Health and Nursing Care.* **1**, 16.

Hood, S., Birnie, D., Swan, L. & Hillis, W. (1998) Questionnaire survey of thrombolytic therapy treatment in accident and emergency departments in the UK. *British Medical Journal.* **316**, 274.

Hugman, R. (1991) *Power in Caring Professions.* Macmillan, London.

ISIS-2 (International Study of Infarct Survival – 2 Collaborative Group (1988) Randomised trial of intravenous streptokinase, oral aspirin, both, or neither among cases of suspected myocardial infarction. *The Lancet.* **2**, 349–360.

Johnson, J. A. & Boss, R. W. (1991) Management development and change in a demanding health care environment. *Journal of Management Development.* **10**, 5–10.

Julian, D. G. (1988) A milestone for myocardial infarction. *British Medical Journal.* **297**, 497–498.

Julian, D. G. (1994) Thrombolysis, the general practitioner and the electrocardiogram. *British Heart Journal.* **72**, 220–221.

Kendrick, K. (1995) Nurses and doctors: a problem of partnership. In: *Interprofessional Relations in Health Care* (eds K. Soothill, L. Mackay & C. Webb), pp. 239-253. Edward Arnold, London.

Leape, L. L., Brennan, T. A., Laird, N. M., Lawthers, A. G., Localio, A. R., Barnes, B. A., Herbert, L., Newhouse, J. P., Weiler, P. C. & Hiatt, H. (1991) The nature of adverse events in hopsitalized patients. Results of the Harvard Medical Practice study II. *New England Journal of Medicine.* **324**, 377–384.

MacKay, L. (1993) *Conflicts in Care, Medicine and Nursing.* Chapman & Hall, London.

McCabe, M. & West, R. (1998) Time to thrombolysis in acute myocardial infarction, in a representative sample of 30 UK hospitals. *Coronary Health Care.* **2**, 81–83.

Mitchell, G. (1997) Reengineered healthcare: why nurses matter. *Nursing Science Quarterly.* **10**, 70–71.

NMC (2002) *Code of Professional Conduct.* Nursing & Midwifery Council, London.

Pell, A., Miller, H. C., Robertson, C. & Fox, K. (1992) Effects of 'Fast Track' admission for acute myocardial infarction on delay to thrombolysis. *British Medical Journal.* **304**, 83–87.

Quinn, T. (1995) Can nurses safely assess suitability for thrombolytic therapy? A pilot study. *Intensive and Critical Care Nursing.* **11**, 126–129.

Rawles, J. (1997) Quantification of the benefit of earlier thrombolytic therapy: five year results of the Grampian region early antistreplase trial (GREAT). *Journal of the American College of Cardiology.* **30**, 1181–1186.

Ryan, T., Anderson, J., Antman, E. & Branniff, B. (1997) Guidelines of the management of patients with acute myocardial infarction: a report of the

American College of Cardiology/American Heart Association Task Force on Practice Guidelines. *Journal of the American College of Cardiology.* **28**, 1328–1428.

Somauroo, J. D., McCarten, P., Appleton, B., Amadi, A. & Rodrigues, E. (1999) Effectiveness of a 'thrombolysis nurse' in shortening delay to thrombolysis in acute myocardial infarction. *Journal of Royal College of Physicians.* **33**, 46–50.

Stein, E. I. (1967) The doctor–nurse game. *Archives of General Psychiatry.* **16**, 699–703.

Stein, L. T., Watts, D. T. & Howell, T. (1990) The doctor–nurse game revisited. *Nursing Outlook.* **38**, 264–268.

Sweet, S. J. & Norman, I. J. (1995) The nurse–doctor relationship: a selective literature review. *Journal of Advanced Nursing.* **22**, 165–170.

Thiemann, D. R., Coresh, J., Schulman, S. P., Gerstenblith, G., Oetgen, W. J., Powe, N. R. (2000) Lack of benefit for intravenous thrombolysis in patients with myocardial infarction who are older than 75 years. *Circulation.* **101**, 2239–2246.

Underhill, S. L., Woods, S. L., Sivarajan Froelicher, E. S. & Halpenny, C. J. (1990) *Cardiovascular Medications for Cardiac Nursing.* Lippincott Company, Philadelphia.

UKCC Midwifery & Health Visiting (1996) *Transitional Arrangements. Specialist practitioner title/ specialist qualification.* United Kingdom Central Council for Nursing, London.

Vincent, C., Neale, G. & Woloshynowych, M. (2001) Adverse events in British hospitals: preliminary retrospective record review. *British Medical Journal.* **322**, 517–519.

Walsh, M. (2000) *Nursing Frontiers: Accountability and the boundaries of care.* Butterworth Heinemann, Oxford.

Walsh, M. & Ford, P. (1990) *Nursing Rituals: Research and rational action.* Heinemann Nursing, Oxford.

Watson, J. (1998) *Nursing: Human Science and Human Care. A theory of nursing.* National League for Nursing, New York.

Watson, J. (1999) *Postmodern Nursing and Beyond.* Churchill Livingstone, London.

Westwood, P. J. & Prosser S. M. (1997) Evaluation of a critical care pathway to reduce the door-to-needle times for thrombolytic therapy following a myocardial infarction. *Coronary Health Care.* **1**, 200–205.

Wilson, R., Runciman, W. B., Gibberd, R. W., Harrison, B. T., Newby, L. & Hamilton, J. D. (1995) The Quality in Australian Health Care study. *Medical Journal of Australia.* **163**, 458–471.

# 10. *Talking Harm, Whispering Death – An Exploration of Iatrogenic Harm in Palliative Care*

*Valerie Young*

**Editors' note**

> This chapter is written in the first person to capture the personal and subjective elements of caring and their impact on professional discourses. The author has changed key parts of the stories included to ensure the anonymity of those people/patients referred to. Although nurses were the co-participants in the research on which this chapter is based, patients' stories abound because nursing discourse often prioritised patients as the central characters around which nurses' own stories of caring develop.

## *Introduction and background*

> Other chapters have explored the unintentional harm inflicted on patients through aspects of clinical diagnosis or treatment. Medical comment and clinical words also cause unintentional harm, and though they don't usually break bones, they hurt and have the potential to break lives. It is to the dimension of harm by medical comment that I turn in this chapter where I examine Illich's (1990) notions of cultural and social iatrogenesis within the context of research that I undertook in palliative care settings. I will argue that the time of breaking bad news, the time of turmoil and chaos, is a potential location for nurses in particular to explore alternative ways of expressing caring which transcend the institutionalised norms that so often express themselves in cultural and social iatrogenesis. For example, instead of letting rehearsed words of

palliation deafen the silence of shock, nurses can honour patients' silence and loneliness, and when patients again have a voice, can hear and listen to their needs, and ultimately help de-institutionalise dying.

Because language is culturally and socially shaped and honed, particular attention will be paid to its professional and lay use in the research data. Here, nurses and patients reveal how 'talking harm' emerges from cultural and social practices that mask the inevitability of dying, muffling it in whispers and hushed tones, concealing it behind closed doors of physical institutions and institutionalised minds. However, the co-participants (those nurses who participated in the research) also reveal another voice – the particular and individual voice of nurses and patients – and its attempts to be heard and understood.

According to Ricoeur (1984), when we nurture experience, and articulate it through language, we make the experience become itself: it is by narrating, by telling the story of our experiences and by listening to the stories of others about us that we interpret and understand ourselves. It has been said that we are our stories. By exploring nurses' stories of caring for people in palliative care settings and stories told to them by patients we can inform the ways that professional discourses have shaped the lives of those living their dying. By discourse I mean the way in which professionals organise, prioritise and manage the telling of a particular social and cultural narrative.

For Foucault (1981) discourses are dynamic: knowledge is created through discourse, and discourse produces, resists, undermines and exposes power. The following stories illuminate Foucault's (1981) appreciation that the institutional locations of discourses, such as hospitals and health centres, also harbour others that can reverse the power dynamics and challenge the status quo. In other words, and as discussed in Chapter 2, although a powerful discourse may be operating, e.g. the discourse of western medicine, other discourses have the power to resist and to offer alternatives.

The stories described here were selected from narrative interviews held with 16 qualified nurses (Young, 2000). Prior to the interviews appropriate ethical approval and consent were gained from the nurses who were informed that aspects of the research would, were this possible and appropriate, be published. Anonymity of these research co-participants, and the people/patients to which they refer, has been ensured through the use of pseudonyms and by altering key details. The findings cannot be attributed to any particular geographical area as the co-participants worked in a number of discrete boroughs encompassing many NHS Trusts. The selection of the co-participants stories was purposive and draws on Chambers' notion of presenting them as the oppositional practice of resistance to professional discourses that shape western health care practice (Chambers, 1991). I do not wish to undermine professional discourse but to draw attention to some of its limitations and to the harm caused by assumption of its greatness. Western medicine and its appropriation by allied professions continues to obscure and take over the power of individuals to heal themselves when dying (Illich, 1990), and to take from them their ability to create or continue their own life stories (Hunt, 1992). However, this chapter concludes that when medical discourse is articulated with personal and potential nursing discourses, the ability to heal when dying can be redeemed.

## The people

Mary's story draws attention to the nature of narrative. Narrative is an important concept in this chapter and will be defined according to its traditional and contemporary understandings. Mary's story draws attention to the claims that a grand-narrative (traditional interpretation of narrative) makes on someone's life. As well as carrying meaning, words carry power relationships. These relationships are exposed by practitioners and patients who explore the ways in which untimely and unreflective words of health care professionals silence patients' words and fill the space around dying with rehearsed commentary that sounds hollow and is stripped of authenticity.

Dying people are problematic to contemporary living. They destabilise efforts to curtail and deny death. To a great extent medicine and nursing maintain the illusion of the permanence of life by fragmenting dying into different medical challenges and social projects that portray death as inhuman. Manifestations of dying are shrouded in curative language and technologies. Dying people are veiled behind screens and in hospital side-rooms. Offensive dying is hidden from public view in hospices and nursing homes (Lawton, 1998); even dying at home can be strictly controlled and normalised (Hunt, 1992; Hart *et al.*, 1998). Social iatrogenic harm (Illich, 1990) extends the physical dislocation and geographical relocation of dying people to an existential dislocation too: people who are dying can find that natural changes associated with dying and their wholeness when dying are dismantled into diverse, treatable, palliative and in the case of visible signs of dying, into maskable events.

However, I wish to validate the need for a medical discourse. Medical discourse is necessary but its one-sidedness needs to be recognised and challenged. Although the stories shared here explain the necessity of the objective knowledge inherent in a medical discourse, they also suggest the need for its articulation in conjunction with the subjective experiences of illness, and with the artistry (aesthetics) and ethical relationships that comprise caring. It is possible that professional carers, nurses for example, who could articulate these discourses, instead frequently mirror a medical stance.

Becci's story (which like the others cited here is described by the palliative care nurse that worked with her) explores how nurses might help patients to reintegrate a sense of who they are as people (self), not just patients. Becci's experience draws attention to an interesting paradox. It demonstrates that although professional words and commentary are powerful, patients' usually are not. In considering patients' medical histories, the visual, in Becci's case the power of the written text, endures and presides over the spoken word: the assumed objectivity of clinical vision overwhelms the patient's voice. Stories about Susan and Tara follow this theme. They reverberate with the power of the voice of medicine. When the voice of medicine drowns the personal voice it also strips the illness experience of its subjective, biographical content to make it abstract, context free and consistent with a powerful, scientific discourse. Tara screamed out her individuality but her subjectivity had to compete with the objectivity of medicine, which was so immersed in its dogma that it could not hear Tara.

The prior lives of people – their biographies, their dreams – do not die once people become ill or once told that their predicted life spans are limited by illness. Neither must people's lives necessarily be torn apart by the diagnosis of a very serious illness. Peter's story illuminates how the aesthetic of caring, the skill and craft of being in tune with the patient's narrative, allows professionals to overcome bias to ensure a dignified dying experience that honours individual lives. Peter's story is one that challenges our cultural assumptions that serious illness is disruptive, and that patients labelled 'loners' require benevolent or parental type care.

The chapter ends with Jessica's story. This is a graphic portrayal of Jessica's reintegration of her sense of self. Its placement in a medical discourse renders its resistance (Chambers, 1991) all the more poignant and powerful. Jessica's story not only challenges the privilege of any particular narrative but also indicates the complexity of dying in a society that has such difficulty in enabling space to imagine and prepare for dying.

## Medicine's grand-narrative

It seems that once a person becomes a patient they are in danger of having their lives rewritten, not by themselves but by professionals who may silence their words, and replace their story with a medical grand-narrative concurring with that of a classical narrative structure.

### Defining narrative

A narrative is the shape and plot of a story. Narratives are structured by the prevalent discourse of the time, i.e. the way a particular profession manages and prioritises different characters and particular events to shape a particular story. A clear example is in the way that traditional history books are written. Women are practically absent in history: their contribution to local and world events is all but absent from most history books to the extent that many adults are unaware of women's historical roles. In the classic narrative, events in the story follow a basic structure from problem to resolution. At the beginning of the story an event may take place to disrupt a person's equilibrium or the meaning or significance the person holds in his or her family and society. It is then a task of the characters, plot and process to resolve the disruption and restore equilibrium (Barthes, 1977). The difficulty of this narrative structure becomes apparent when the enigma is cancer and narrative structure is supposed to organise a cure. The patient's dying breaks the rules of the ideal medical narrative that is premised on cure rather than on failure to cure. Of course when the story is fictional, miracles often occur. Explorations of real-life narratives, however, reveal that in western culture the story can be usurped by medicine, recharacterising the person who has cancer as a patient. For example patienthood sometimes fragments personhood (Goffman, 1976; Gadow 1980) because of its tendency to confront the sick person with an object interior body. This is a body that has previously been integrated with one's sense of self, a body that has been taken for granted but which now asserts an authority or a threat to selfhood. That body is now explored as a physical object rather than being integrated with a subjective person, a body that the patient may begin to perceive as alien.

Ultimately, to comply with a sanitised social tolerance of death when death cannot be protracted, the patient's life is often replotted in a medical script that prescribes the person's dying trajectory in a cultural biography (Hunt, 1992). This is acceptable if it is the patient's choice. But we need to question the tension between patient choice, collusion with and dominance by a classical medical narrative.

## Defining cultural iatrogenesis

Illich (1990, p. 42) says this of cultural iatrogenesis:

> '... the so-called health professions have an even deeper, culturally health-denying effect in so far as they destroy the potential of people to deal with their human weakness, vulnerability and uniqueness in a personal and autonomous way.... This cultural iatrogenesis ... is the ultimate backlash of hygienic progress and consists in the paralysis of healthy responses to suffering, impairment, and death.'

Illich accepts that illness and dying are integral to human existence although difficult to accept within a society that seeks to minimise pain and discomfort. The significance of his observations will be addressed later in the chapter.

## *Imposing a medical narrative*

### Mary's story

Mary fought the grand-narrative of medicine in order to reclaim her own dying narrative but she was often thwarted. Mary was in her late forties and had been something of a medical success story having lived the last decade and a half of her life cured of cancer. Unfortunately, following some later tests, her general practitioner (GP) told her that she now had disseminated carcinoma and should 'take it on the chin' (Young, 2000). The district nurse visited Mary at her GP's request. Mary found herself being compelled into a medical narrative structure that recharacterised her as a patient whose continued life trajectory would be dependent on medicine and whose uniqueness as a person was unlikely to be recognised. The ending of her story had already been timed. Now her district nurse set out her narrative trajectory of the rest of her life in an institutionalising discourse of confinement and finality. She warned that she would be there at the beginning and there at the end. She predicted the deterioration of Mary's autonomy and control, warning her that she would need a pressure mattress and would probably need hospice care for symptom control. Okri cautions us against the use of such unreflective words and warns of their power.

> 'It sometimes seems to me that our days are poisoned with too many words. Words said and not meant. Words said and meant. Words divorced from feeling. Wounding words. Words that conceal. Words that reduce. Dead words' (Okri, 1997 p. 88).

Mary, a fiercely independent woman, was terrified by the pattern that was unfolding in these words. She refused to see the district nurse again. However, despite her feistiness, by the time her friend persuaded her to see a Macmillan Nurse (a specialist nurse practitioner in palliative care) three weeks later, the story of the rest of Mary's life was already being restructured according to the powerful medical narrative. During her initial interview with her Macmillan Nurse she said that she had given her favourite clothes away. She was being ushered along the collective grand-narrative by the powerful impact of her medical prognosis. However, she continued to feel well. She lived for a further eighteen months. Ironically, when it became apparent that she would outlive her prognosis, she told her Macmillan Nurse that she longed for the beautiful velvet scarf that she had given to her friend. When her nurse suggested that she should treat herself to another she retorted that she had of course given all her money away (Young, 2000; 2002).

Mary the *patient* was not given permission to be Mary the *person* who possibly had the internal and external resources to remain outside the patient role. She was not given time to consider the meaning of her diagnosis within her own lived experience. Before she could even contemplate the meaning of her illness, she was told that she should take it on the chin. She had difficulty in planning her own journey towards dying because her non-compliance did not fit within an ideal patient characterisation. Had Mary's personhood been allowed to feature in the story, albeit controlled within a medical narrative, she might have felt able to participate. But promises of being there at the beginning and there at the end required her compliance rather than participation. The harm caused by the expectation that a patient should succumb to the medical narrative was complicated by its power to marginalise Mary. She still needed help but wished it in terms of who she was as a person with all her strengths and vulnerabilities, rather than according to a prescription of patienthood.

The impasse between Mary and her general practice team was played out in a Foucauldian power dynamic: she continued to challenge their attempts to prescribe how she should conduct her life, which culminated in sanctions such as the failure of the services to lend Mary's family a commode. Such actions were achieved by the use of delaying tactics and a lack of response to voicemail requests for assistance by Mary's family at the terminal stages of her cancer. They contributed to her husband's ultimate decision to buy the private services of a palliative care nurse because he feared being let down again by the local health services.

The irony of stories like Mary's is that though the prevailing discourse is death-denying, it is apparent that when professionals can no longer deny that they are unable to cure, the patient is projected into a linear and hierarchical medical narrative of dying that makes it very difficult for them to carve out a space for living the way they desire to live while preparing to die the way they desire.

## Shattered living and shattered dying

The opportunity of finding space to grow when dying is often curtailed in western society. In exploring how 22 staff nurses defined and interpreted their work with terminally ill patients, May (1995) identified a serious contradiction in nurses' work. Although sensitive to the importance of nurse–patient talk, and sensitive to the importance of listening to patients when bad news had been broken, nurses nevertheless curtailed patient responses. He says: '... nurses' accounts reveal an order and predictability to the forms of work which they mobilize in the period in which the patient is coming to terms with this bad news' (May, 1995 p. 558). Other researchers (Hunt, 1992; Lawton, 1999) acknowledged the discourse of the social in the ways hospitals and hospices establish a regular and routine pattern of death. Although nurses may feel they are being spontaneous in their response, they are frequently repeating aspects of the medical discourse with which they are so familiar.

### Defining social iatrogenesis

Illich (1990, p. 41) suggests that social iatrogenesis is at work

'... when health care is turned into a standardized item, a staple; when all suffering is "hospitalized" and homes become inhospitable to birth, sickness, and death; when the language in which people could experience their bodies is turned into bureaucratic gobbledegook; or when suffering, mourning and healing outside the patient role are labelled a form of deviance".

In a study of patients dying at home, Hunt (1992) revealed that even when at home, the dying and their families followed a medical script. Rather than creating their own dying trajectory, patients tended to dismiss individualistic 'scripts' or those that might contradict those of their professional carers. Hunt felt that patients were inclined to espouse the wishes of their nurses to the extent of covering up anger and fear of dying. Even in their own homes, patients' deaths were sanitised and normalised to fit the good death desired by others (Hunt, 1992; Hart *et al.*, 1998). There are alternatives. Community nurses do, for example, resist the convenient relocation of bedroom to downstairs living/dying room. Some nurses break with tradition by doing everything to maintain the intimacy of family relationships and spaces. Closeness between parents and children or husband and wife is paramount to these carers who define the 'good death' as the death desired and determined by those who are dying.

In the sociological literature the discourse of 'shattered lives' is most closely articulated within the theory of 'biographical disruption' (Bury 1982, 2001). Bury's work, based on qualitative research on the emerging impact of rheumatoid arthritis on a group of relatively young women and men, identified that much of the distress relating to diagnosis was due to its imagery as a disease of the elderly. Bury (2001) recognised, however, that patients' living with chronic illness can contest biomedical narratives of illness with personal narratives because of the increase in incidence and public recognition of chronic illnesses. It helps that signs of some chronic illnesses are transient and can be hidden from public view. Yet, when we compare this biographical disruption and its imagery with the disruption of dying, we can recognise the absence of an imagery of dying in what has become our death-denying society. Bauman (1998, p. 220) says:

'We may comment: the corollary of the 'disenchantment of death', the resolute modern refusal to 'think through death', the decision to exile it to the margins of awareness together with everything else which has been proclaimed unknown and unknowable, and the related suppression of death-fright – is the dispersion of the issue of mortality...'

Phrases like 'I'm here at the beginning, I'll be here at the end' rush into the disruption. The words and phrases sound hollow because they are not about the person who is dying, they are about delaying and fragmenting the hold of death,

> '. . . dismantling it then becomes the joint obligation of the medical profession and the population whose mode of living it now scripts, monitors and supervises.'

Bauman, 1998 p. 221

## *To see a voice: the struggle between personal and professional discourses*

### Susan's story

Susan had cancer. She also had cancer spots on several parts of her body and developed problems because of secondary cancer. She had severe nausea and vomiting and was therefore admitted to a surgical ward for investigations. Initially the cause was difficult to identify. She looked unwell. During the consultant's ward round she told him how awful she felt and explained that she had already vomited five times that day. In the absence of medical evidence and, one assumes, the consultant's ability to appreciate Susan's predicament, he said, 'I only have your word for it'. It seems that Susan's word meant nothing and her planned exploratory surgery was cancelled. Wendell (1996) points out that the vocabulary of illness is a third-person scientific and quasi-scientific description, which is inadequate for both medical practitioners and patients. Sontag (2001), who also suffered from advanced cancer, complained at the difficulty she had in articulating and interpreting her illness because of the limited vocabulary available to her. In science, the sense of vision is perceived to be more objective, pure and detached than that of voice and hearing (Belenky *et al.*, 1997; Rée, 1999) which are perceived to be closer, more intimate and related to each other and consequently less reliable.

Susan was operated on only when her symptoms eventually became visible to her professional carers. In theatre she was found to have a tumour wrapped around and obstructing her bowel. Rée (1999) draws attention to the impossibility of valuing one sense, in the above case – vision, and its apprehension of the world over another as we do not really perceive the world through our five separate senses, but with our bodies as a whole. Susan felt unwell in herself and we can appreciate that attempts to speak concerns about our health, to speak concerns derived from our 'bodies as a whole', are limited by the language we must use in doing so.

The veneration of medicine produces a different discourse than other sciences. Wendell (1996) again says that the medical discourse of heroism blames the disease or the person with the disease rather than accepting limitations and blame itself. 'If any healing science or art is believed to have full knowledge and control of the body, then only the individual players – patient and doctor/healer – can be blamed when things go out of control' (Wendell, 1996 p. 129).

## Becci

During her outpatients' appointment Becci told the consultant that the ascites around her stomach and the lymphoedema on her legs were uncomfortable. Her legs were weeping. She had known her body as slim and petite and now she looked pregnant and needed to buy bigger sized clothes. His reply was that he'd seen worse. His words silenced hers. Later she told her community nurse that she was afraid to complain about her symptoms in case he might take her off the clinical trial. So far Becci's cancer had not responded to treatment and she was on a clinical trial that was researching the use of a new drug for the treatment of this type of cancer.

Becci believed that the clinical trial was her only hope and therefore felt powerless, and at her consultant's mercy. Her palliative care nurse helped her explore her feelings about her body. She was so embarrassed in front of her boys. They were teenagers and here she was with one of her breasts all distended and her stomach out like a balloon. It appeared to her nurse that because she was apparently perceived by her consultant as a control subject in his clinical trial, and may have been receiving placebo medication, her symptoms were not important, not acknowledged. Quill & Cassel (1995) elucidate the limbo-land of palliative care patients involved in clinical trials. They suggest that inclusion of palliative care patients in clinical trials may be a way of keeping the focus of the medical profession on the patient who fears abandonment. This requires more research because it is also possible that the repercussions of medicine's unease with failure to cure means that someone like Becci could feel displaced when cure was no longer an option. Becci's involvement in a clinical trial, for example, meant that she was unlikely to be discharged from the cancer centre that offered hope of a cure, no matter how tentative.

The palliative care nurse talked through the alternatives with Becci. In the end Becci decided to write her symptoms down. She read it all out to her consultant when she next saw him; how the ascites was a huge problem for her because her clothes did not fit; her distress at trying to manage her weeping legs; her poor body image, and her discomfort in front of the boys. He listened to her written words, and then he helped her manage the symptoms. And she said that she felt like a person again rather than a die in a gambling game (Young, 2000). Becci to some extent had been fragmenting herself in her fearful effort to fit a narrative structure that she felt was part of the contract but written in the small print.

Following that appointment her consultant remarked on being taken aback at her level of preparation for the interview. He was impressed. I cannot claim by this incident alone that the written, the visible, means more than the oral. However, the integration of Becci's voice in a written text made a difference. The integration of her voice with her nurse's professional knowledge made a difference. The incident draws attention to issues of vision and voice. Belenky *et al.* (1997) suggest that scientists conducting a trial try to approach it blind by distancing themselves from the particular and the intimate. Could this have accounted for the consultant's generalised response to Becci's first attempt to speak of her symptoms? However, in view of Becci's sense of her precarious position between hope and despair, she may possibly have spoken quietly at first lest she spoil the odds.

## Visualising and voicing self: integrating discourses

### Tara

Tara is a medical consultant. She is angry with her medical colleagues who objectively tell her that she knows that she is dying. Tara does know that she is dying but she does not feel that she is dying right now. Her Macmillan Nurse asked her how she wished her medical colleagues to talk about her dying. Her answer was so simple, she said that they could soften their words by saying that they think she is dying, or that they are sorry but feel that she is dying. However, she sensed that their words were clipped, and dehumanised by their clinical presentation. Tara needed to hear caring and hope in their words. She felt that she was not ready to move into the dying space that they opened in front of her. She knew she would probably have to go there soon but her spirit was buoyant right now. She said that they never asked her how she was feeling.

Tara said that her medical colleague's body language told her that he was unable to engage in any emotional discussion about her death. Researchers have drawn attention to the difficulties that professional carers have in maintaining the therapeutic emotional boundaries between self and others (Gadow, 1980; Morse 1991; Wuest, 1998). Morse presents a continuum that moves between disengagement at one pole to overinvolvement at the other. Wuest (1998) suggests that little has been written about the need for establishing limits to caring and my own work re-affirms this (Young, 2000). I recollect the earlier comment from Rée suggesting that we perceive the world through our bodies as a whole. Professional carers do not easily attend to their embodied knowledge, particularly to their personal and aesthetic ways of knowing. The stories already shared in this chapter are evidence of tendencies to separate the professional by disembodying and distancing it from personal, ethical relations, aesthetic and reflective practice. Moreover, these same professionals are more likely to attend to visual objective knowledge with its masculine ethics of impartial justice (Irigaray, 1985; Bauman, 1993).

However, nurse and feminist researchers draw attention to relational ethics, meaning ethics based on the lived experience of being involved with patients (Irigaray, 1985; Gadow, 1989; Watson, 1999). Gadow (1989) explored the necessary subjectivity and embodiment of this relationship in her discussion of nurses' ability to be advocates for silent patients, patients who cannot express their wishes. By attending to the embodied, whole relationship, their feelings, their proximity to patients, the intimacy of physical caring for silent patients, the nurse and patient relate. The nurse embodies the sensitivity and authenticity of the patient and learns to speak for her or him because of being with her or him. Relational ethics expands knowledge from the cognitive of empiric, objective and professional to incorporate emotional, spiritual, aesthetic and embodied ways of being with patients (Gadow, 1989; Rée, 1999; Watson, 1999; Zohar & Marshal, 2001). It is not masculine alone, not feminine alone, but is both relational and androgynous in that it encompasses the nurse's experiences of the scientific and objective and the concrete, sensual and subjective, the feminine and masculine of caring.

At the same time however, Gadow (1980) stresses that when patients recognise their object bodies, they need professionals to recognise the object, clinical body by addressing and describing the illness in language that is disembodied and abstract – by means of a clinical gaze. However, her work points to timeliness of objectivity in that there is a right time to attend to the object body or the general ways that certain illnesses manifest on people in general. She explains that, until the occurrence of illness, people tend to be unconscious of their object selves. It is true to say that healthy and respected individuals are unlikely to be aware of the object body, although some, particularly the oppressed and abused, are accustomed to perceiving their bodies as objects. Timely explanation of its objectivity in general terms is important to help patients understand the cleft that suddenly occurs between self and body, especially during illness. However, Gadow's work stresses the importance of subjective knowledge and the need to reintegrate the object body with one's sense of self as a whole person. It seems that practitioners do not always facilitate and honour this reintegration.

## Jessica

Jessica, a young mother, did not have a communicative relationship with her husband. Now that she had cancer she found that he distanced himself even more. He seemed unable to be involved in the emotional aspects of her illness. On this particular occasion, Jessica, hoping to increase her husband's involvement and his understanding of her as a person living with cancer, asked him to accompany her to her outpatients' appointment. Having been examined by the consultant she was lying on the couch waiting for his evaluation when she suddenly became aware of her object body. She saw herself as she reclined there framed, as though in a painting, while her husband and consultant sat upright, facing each other, talking scientifically about X-rays, the disease and its pathology. Neither of them acknowledged her, or acknowledged that she was the person with the disease about which they spoke. Jessica was angry because the encounter promoted her husband's notion that this disease had nothing to do with her, it was just a general disease. The encounter, the detached discussion between the two men, what Jessica called men's talk, reinforced her husband's emotional distance. At this stage of her life's work, Jessica had reintegrated her body with cancer with her sense of self and was trying to re-engage her husband in her changed life. However, he and the doctor engaged in an objective, medical vocabulary that simultaneously disengaged them from Jessica as the person who had this cancer about which they talked.

## *The not-knowing stance: integrating dying with living*

Newman (1994), a nurse theorist, says that each of us on some occasion in life is brought to a point where the old rules and what we considered to be progress don't work any more. At this juncture we need to learn to transcend a situation that is very difficult in order to find a new way of relating to things and to discover the freedom that comes with overcoming former limitations. The necessity of hanging on in there in the chaos, in the ambiguity and the uncertainty of the situation, is an important factor in the healing process. Newman would explain the healing process as the ability to accept the fact that one is dying and to integrate the notion of death into one's life. Yet the sacredness of the space that might facilitate this and its creative potential are so easily undermined or obscured in the professional hurry to intervene and to resolve the problem for the profession and for society by re-establishing equilibrium.

In contrast to professional responses based in classical narratives, Anderson and Goolishian (1992, p. 28) emphasise a different response based on 'not-knowing'. Not-knowing is a philosophical stance that attempts to challenge privileged standpoints for understanding. It is a stance that appreciates the interpretative, changing nature of understanding. A 'not-knowing' stance challenges fixed scripts and props that sanitise, control and curtail communication around dying for example. Not-knowing involves openness to difference and imagination that integrates an understanding of subjective dying with compassionate professionalism.

In any event Newman cautions that we cannot assume the organised pattern (the one that precedes the period of uncertainty, illness or pain) to be satisfactory and the chaotic pattern to be unsatisfactory. She holds that they are both part of the same process of evolution – of life development and growth. Illness can in fact lead to an expanded consciousness, or a level of functioning that is better than, more developed, and more reflective than previous ways of being. She says:

> 'We as nurses enter into this process with a client to be present with it, attend to it and live it, even if it appears in the form of disharmony, catastrophe, or disease.'
>
> Newman, 1994 p. 99

In a similar vein, Anderson and Goolishian (1992) say that therapeutic conversation is a communion between patient and therapist towards a new narrative because the professional's role, expertise and emphasis is to develop a free conversational space and to facilitate an emerging conversational process in which this 'newness' can occur. Taylor (1994) reminds us of professional responsibility to encompass the ordinary. She says that nursing is human and ordinary and that humanity enables a way to enter into other people's stories and be in their scripts rather than assume that we need to draw people into our professional scripts. However, the point at which palliative care work begins – this turbulent whirlpool or chaotic chasm – is also the point where medical comment can in its haste overlook this uncomfortable turmoil and disharmony. It too easily fills the space with a ready-made performance, a dying trajectory that fits our death-denying culture, one that is constructed as a hygienic mask that sanitises and controls death in a performance, in rehearsed words and sentences.

## Peter's story

Medical words silenced Peter too. On meeting him for the first time his Macmillan Nurse asked him to tell her about his understanding of his illness. In remembering his diagnosis he said that the GP read aloud to him from his notes but he could not understand the words. He said that he thought they must have been medical words but could not understand their meaning. When the GP looked Peter straight in the eye and said that they would do what they could to prolong his life, he realised the import of his words (Young, 2000).

Peter then looked at the Macmillan Nurse, and pre-empted their talk of cancer by saying that he did not like that word. She replied: 'If you don't like using that word what word would you like to use?' In a more confident voice he said that the word tumour did not seem so frightening (Young, 2002). Although Peter also chose a clinical terminology, he felt comfortable with this. Peter's Macmillan Nurse was aware that Peter's insular life and his sparse home broke the norm expected for home deaths. His eccentricity marked out difference, difference that could mar support. His passion for his garden, its view and nature that surrounded him also indicated the inhospitality of the confines of a hospital ward to Peter's dying.

Peter asked if he could still go to the pub now that he had cancer. Mary had previously asked if she could continue to be involved in the townswomen's guild. Though on the one hand both Mary and Peter attempted to construct their individual stories in their own words, on the other they gave evidence that their intuitive grasp on their own lives was disrupted. Peter also asked what was expected of people in his position. In particular he asked if the expectation was that he should commit suicide. Mary and Peter revealed vulnerability, a weakness in their storyline that could be shattered by that of the ready-made story of the medicalised, clinical dying trajectory waiting to be shaped for them in both cultural and social iatrogenesis. That medical journey included for them a possible withdrawal from the everyday events of a pre-terminally ill life.

This is a difficult time for the person who is ill and for professionals who are informing them of their illness and trying to support them. Theorists (Watson, 1999; Zohar & Marshall, 2001) and patients suggest to me that this yearning, this void, this bio-graphical disruption itself may be better off left a while, the space acknowledged and tolerated. It seems that the answer does not come in the sanitised and hygienic mask of a medical dramaturgy, the word coined by Goffman to describe the performative nature of responses and reassurances, or I would suggest the ready-made social script that is so readily offered. Perhaps the answer comes in what May & Fleming (1997) call 'professional imagination', a nursing attitude and way of being with patients that honour the dynamic and co-creational scope of both in that encounter. Watson (1985) called this a *transpersonal caring moment* that expands beyond the moment: '... the process goes beyond itself, and becomes part of the life history of each person, as well as part of the larger, deeper complex pattern of life' (Watson, 1985 p. 59).

In focusing on the lived experiences of caring relationships, this embracing narrative configures the professional imagination. It is reflexive in that it recognises and challenges the grand-narrative of medicine as well as the personal and institutional narrative discussed in this chapter.

## Space and time: the gift relationship

Peter was at home in his own environment but would not easily be at home in another. Though Zohar and Marshall (2001) recognise the dilemmas of health care professionals caring for dying people, they urge us to speak spontaneously rather than in practised lines. They suggest that health care professionals need courage, power and strength to emerge from behind their clinical masks, particu-larly when patients are very vulnerable. Their recognition of pro-fessional defensiveness is explored by Lindseth *et al.* (1994) in their study of nurses' and physicians' reflections on their narratives about ethically difficult care episodes. Their work suggests that when practitioners are in difficult situations they tend to perceive the story in which they are now participating, or about to be involved, as negative or bad. Lindseth *et al.* (1994 p. 243) draw on the notion of spontaneity to liberate practitioners from this defen-sive position that fosters curtailment of conversation and commu-nication.

'The utterances of life are spontaneous; that is, they work best when we do not have to think about them.'

Lindseth *et al.*, 1994 p. 245

The authors explain that professional practitioners are inclined to feel a breakdown in their own trustworthiness and sympathy when breaking bad news to patients. Consequently, the news is more likely to be broken in a way that is formal and rehearsed than spontaneous.

The nurse caring for Peter was intuitive in their relationship. She planned Peter's care in terms of his individuality. She worked both spontaneously and reflectively with Peter. She had found a hospice with open spaces, a beautiful garden and views, all of which were so important to Peter. Anticipating that Peter's particular cancer, metastatic carcinoma involving the lower part of his neck and upper chest, would ultimately need very skilled symptom control, together they planned his final days in the hospice which they visited while he was well. In the final days of Peter's life he made his way to the outpatient department. His consultant, who appreciated Peter's sense of place, confirmed that it was now time to go to the hospice. Peter asked to return home to be in his garden one last time. Though he struggled to breathe, his consultant supported his request and his Macmillan Nurse helped him to make this journey and watched him take in the beauty of his landscape. Later, though very breathless he wanted to walk into the hospice rather than be wheeled in by wheelchair. She physically supported this very important journey too (Young, 2000).

Consideration of the potential harm of habitual use of rehearsed lines and performances challenges the ways many practitioners work. Reflection is more than contemplation, assimilation of past experiences into a repertoire for the future, or a self-rejoinder to avoid a particular action in the future. Reflective practitioners need to be dynamic, questioning their tendencies to bank useful and routine responses, which can undermine reflexivity. Generally though, reflection even at its most imaginative calls on the past to help manage the present and anticipate the future. But Løgstrup (1983) (cited in Lindseth *et al.*, 1994) warns that not all of caring can call on the past. Being present means just that, 'presencing'. It demands risk, imagination and spontaneity and the courage to use tacit skills that tend to emerge in relation with patients, in the energy and aesthetics of the space that is there and which both patient and carer together occupy at a particular moment. My own experiences and my readings of others tell me that spontaneity can be about recognising, honouring someone's loneliness and isolation by being consciously silent and patient.

Mayeroff (1990) says that presence, presencing, the dynamic energy of the practitioner's true presence with the patient, collapses space and time together, enlarging both. Fox (1998) talks about nomadism, similar to 'not-knowing', as a presence that is multiple, changing, open, where individuals can be different. The difference, even though fleeting, opens a space for dying that offers some freedom from culturally and socially inhibiting narratives, freedom to die according to the way one might wish to die. He says that nomadism demands the courage to contest 'the patterning of subjectivity' which discourses normally require. It is a 'gift relationship' with others defined by their otherness rather than being redefined to accord with a certain discursive norm.

## Conclusion

Whispering death – death that is whispered rather than talked about clearly and truthfully – provokes tension, inhibition, distortion and curtailment in talk that harms. Medical comment is important because people at times require the objectivity of the clinical gaze and the practical help it might offer. However, medical and nursing care require more than this objectivity and detachment. The task for professional carers is to be able to integrate medical discourse within a compassionate professionalism that acknowledges both the limits of medicine and the infinity of the imagination. Although it is evident that some nurses expand the notion of professional narrative to include compassion, empathy and relationship, many restrict it to its narrowest expression, the mimicry of medicine. There are moments in the above stories that reveal how easily patients and families too who have no imagery of dying in a society that denies death, gaze blinkered through the distancing lens offered by medical narrative because they know of no other.

Reflection on nurses' management of patients' dying underscores possibilities that might reduce harm caused by acculturated and institutionalised medical comment. Although several of the above stories highlight the omnipotence of a certain professionalised narrative that is told, written or lived according to particular conventions, other stories reveal the ways in which this narrative is challenged from within its own professions and from without. Mary's struggle to live and die a good death according to her own and her family's wishes was consistently undermined by an inflexible and linear professional narrative. Peter's story differed in that his individuality and vulnerability were recognised and the medical narrative, rather than being heroic and superior, embraced Peter's and accommodated him in a structure that was able to be flexible and imaginative. Though the language of medicine proved

212

an initial threat, the compassion and empathy of a key professional enabled Peter's voice.

In reviewing this chapter I am struck by a certain contradiction between vision and voice. It seems that talking harm follows a detached gaze: when practitioners distance themselves from patients by perceiving patients as object bodies only, they are in danger of curtailing their own and patients' subjective voices. The ability to focus more deeply and laterally on the patient as subject and object body requires practitioners to embrace their own subjectivity. Talking healing rather than harm requires the voice of compassion and empathy. Yes, it requires scientific knowledge and clinical competence but these are lenses for looking at parts of the body, not the whole person. Medical comment needs to emerge from relationship with self, with profession and with patients. It is a voice that resonates and synchronises when it integrates being, doing and knowing, rather than taking up the banner of a single dimension.

## Reducing harm in palliative care

In order to minimise unnecessary harm in palliative care those working in health care might:

i.   reflect on their own understandings of the aim of palliative care
ii.  develop a professional discourse that challenges and expands that of medicine rather than unreflectively and partially mirrors or mimics it
iii. recognise and honour patient strengths and vulnerabilities to harness these to facilitate continuation and expansion of patient and family living when dying
iv.  develop knowledge of the power and potential of professional/ patient relationship.

## *Author's note*

I wish to acknowledge the contribution of my friend and colleague Deirdre Watkins to this work. Her insights as a Clinical Nurse Specialist and storyteller have been invaluable.

## *References*

Anderson, H. & Goolishian, H. (1992) The client is the expert: a not-knowing approach to therapy. In: *Therapy as Social Construction* (eds S. McNamee & K.Gergen), pp. 25–39. Sage, New York.

Barthes, R. (1977) *Image–Music–Text.* Fontana, London.

Bauman, Z. (1998) Postmodern adventures of life and death. In: *Modernity, Medicine and Health* (eds J. Scambler & P. Higgs), pp. 216–231. Routledge, London.

Belenky, M., Clinchy, B., Goldberger, N. & Tarule, J. (1997) *Women's Ways of Knowing: The development of self, voice, and mind*, 10th anniversary edition. Basic Books, New York.

Bury, M. R. (1982) Chronic illness as biographical disruption. *Sociology of Health and Illness.* **4**, 167–182.

Bury, M. R. (2001) Illness narratives: fact or fiction? *Sociology of Health and Illness.* **23**, 263–285.

Chambers, R. (1991) *Room for Manoeuvre: Reading (the) oppositional (in) Narrative.* Manchester University Press, Manchester.

Foucault, M. (1981) *A History of Sexuality: An introduction.* Penguin, Harmondsworth.

Fox, N. (1998) The Promise of postmodernism for the sociology of health and medicine. In: *Modernity, Medicine and Health* (eds G. Scambler & P. Higgs), pp. 29–45. Routledge, London.

Gadow, S. (1980) Existential advocacy: philosophical foundation of nursing. In: *Nursing: Image and Ideals* (eds M. F. Prickler & S. Gadow), pp. 79–101. Springer, New York.

Goffman, E. (1976) *The Presentation of Self in Everyday Life.* Pelican Books, Harmondsworth.

Hart, B., Sainsbury, P. & Short, S. (1998) Whose dying? A sociological critique of the 'good death'. *Mortality.* **3**, 65–77.

Hunt, M. (1992) 'Scripts' for dying at home – displayed in nurses', patients' and relatives' talk. *Journal of Advanced Nursing.* **17**, 1297–1302.

Illich, I. (1990) *Limits to Medicine, Medical Nemesis: The expropriation of health.* Penguin Books, London.

Irigaray, L. (1985) *This Sex Which is Not One.* Cornell University Press, New York.

Lawton, J. (1998) Contemporary hospice care: the sequestration of the unbounded body and 'dirty dying'. *Sociology of Health and Illness.* **20**, 121–143.

Lindseth, A. Marhaug, V. Norberg, A. & Udén, G. (1994) Registered nurses' and physicians' reflections on their narratives about ethically difficult care episodes. *Journal of Advanced Nursing.* **20**, 245–250.

May, C. (1995) 'To call it work somehow demeans it': the social construction of talk in the care of terminally ill patients. *Journal of Advanced Nursing.* **22**, 556–561.

May, C. & Fleming C. (1997) The professional imagination: narrative and the symbolic boundaries between medicine and nursing. *Journal of Advanced Nursing.* **25**, 1094–1100.

Mayeroff, M. (1990) *On Caring.* Harper Perennial, New York.

Morse, J. (1991) Negotiating commitment and involvement in the nurse–patient relationship. *Journal of Advanced Nursing.* **16**, 455–466.

Newman, M. (1984) *Health as Expanding Consciousness*. C. V. Mosby, St. Louis.

Okri, B. (1997) *A Way of Being Free*. Phoenix House, London.

Quill, T. & Cassel, C. (1995) Nonabandonment: a central obligation for physicians. *Annals of Internal Medicine*. **122**, 368–374.

Rée, J. (1999) *I See a Voice: Language, deafness and the senses – a philosophical history*. Harper Collins, London.

Ricoeur, P. (1984) *Time and Narrative*. University of Chicago Press, Chicago.

Sontag, S. (2001) *Illness as Metaphor and AIDS and its Metaphors*. Picador USA, New York.

Taylor, B. (1994) *Being Human, an Ordinariness in Nursing*. Churchill Livingstone, Melbourne.

Watson, J. (1985) *Human Science and Human Care*. Reprinted (1999). Jones & Bartlett, Boston.

Watson, J. (1999) *Postmodern Nursing and Beyond*. Churchill Livingstone, London.

Wendell, S. (1996) *The Rejected Body: Feminist philosophical reflections on disability*. Routledge, London.

Wuest, J. (1998) Illuminating environmental influences on women's caring. *Journal of Advanced Nursing*. **26**, 49–58.

Young, V. (2000) Good enough Nursing: an exploration of the ways that nurses negotiate interprofessional relationships in managing critical incidents. Unpublished MSc dissertation, University of Luton, England.

Young, V. (2002) Pieces of time, *Nursing Philosophy*. **3**, 90–103.

Zohar, D. & Marshall, I. (2001) *Spiritual Intelligence: The ultimate intelligence*. Bloomsbury Publishing, London.

# 11. NHS Direct – Reducing Unnecessary Harm in Health Care through Information Technology and Shifting Nurse Roles

*Richard Winter and Stuart Thompson*

## Introduction

The introduction of information technologies has had a significant effect at many levels within health care. However, the use of such technologies in tasks such as health assessment, record keeping and remote access to health information, has until recently been limited in the UK. NHS Direct, a nurse-led telephone health advice and assessment service, is at the leading edge of change in this area of the National Health Service (NHS) combining computer technology with the knowledge of experienced nurses. This chapter outlines the introduction of NHS Direct and attempts to analyse the impact it is having on reducing risk in contemporary health care in the UK. Any such analysis must of course be tentative, as at the time of writing (late 2002), the results of commissioned research are limited.

## The drivers for change

The development of NHS Direct was prompted by both technological and political changes. The development of reliable health assessment software and increasing public acceptance of telephone contact between patient and practitioner made such a system practical. The telephone has become a ubiquitous part of everyday life and has increasingly been used for remote access to a range of services by the public. It was in some ways inevitable that health care would follow this trend. Recent government objectives have aimed to increase accessibility to health care whilst containing costs. The development of NHS Direct was based on two key documents that set out a programme of modernisation for the NHS: *The New NHS, Modern and Dependable* (DoH, 1997), and *A First Class Service* (DoH, 1998). While neither document intended to define all aspects of NHS Direct, they pointed to both increased accessibility to health care and the use of information technology. The documents set the goals to which the government required that the health service would work. Promoting high quality standards of care, accompanied by more expedient assessment and treatment of patients set within a robust clinical governance framework, were key parts of this. The latter is explained in more detail towards the end of the chapter.

The National Health Service Plan (DoH, 2000a) aimed to set out the timetable for modernisation, promoting NHS Direct as a focal access point for health care, complementing aspects of the role undertaken by the general practitioner (GP). Other key objectives of the plan included:

i.   widening access to health care assessment
ii.  offering advice about health related lifestyle choices for all sectors of society including, by 2003, a free nationally available translation and interpretation service
iii. giving people more choice about how they access the NHS
iv.  enhanced development of information technology as part of the infrastructure of the NHS allowing access through the internet, digital TV and NHS Direct information points
v.   the implementation of computerised patient records
vi.  all GP practices to be connected to the NHS Net by 2002 allowing health data to be transferred across the entire health service
vii. the enhancement of integrated care pathways, which are pre-determined care processes, within defined time scales, for patients presenting with health needs which will map out the expected progress of the patient, detailing tasks to be carried out, the correct sequence and timing of these, and specify who should undertake them (see also Campbell *et al.*, 1998).

The NHS Direct information points referred to above consist of a television monitor through which people can access NHS Direct

217

health advice using touch screen technology. By 2004 there will be over 500 of these information points found in places as diverse as hospital foyers through to public libraries.

## What is NHS Direct?

NHS Direct is a nurse-led telephone health advice service providing 24 hour access to health care assessment and health information. It uses experienced nurses because they possess good health assessment skills and have relevant clinical experience. These are particularly important, bearing in mind that telephone consultation may heighten uncertainty as the dynamics of normal conversation are changed when visual cues are absent (McLellan, 1999).

The Department of Health (2001a) identified the following aims for NHS Direct which are intended to help enhance the health of those using NHS services. The aims are to:

i.   provide a confidential, reliable and consistent source of professional advice for the public on health care 24 hours a day so that they can manage many of their problems at home or know where to turn for appropriate care
ii.  provide simple and speedy access to a comprehensive and up to date range of health and health related information
iii. improve quality, increase cost effectiveness and reduce unnecessary demand on other NHS services providing more appropriate response to the needs of the public
iv.  allow professionals to develop their role in enabling patients to be partners in self-care, and to help them focus on those patients for whom their skills are most needed.

The first pilot sites for NHS Direct were introduced in 1997. They were based at Milton Keynes, Newcastle and Preston. Further sites were developed in successive waves, and with the introduction of fourth wave sites toward the end of 2000, almost all of England and Wales had access to NHS Direct. There are currently two types of health information sites. They have been designated as Type A and Type B. Type A sites are able to handle more common health information enquiries, while Type B sites are able to deal with a full range of health information enquiries. This includes the more complex queries, which may involve information in regard to specialist subjects such as genetic disorders. This expertise is not available at all NHS Direct sites. Calls are referred to a Type B site when necessary.

Giving the public accurate evidence based health information should enhance their health and the appropriate use of the health service. The ease of access to health information influences positive lifestyle choices and enables the caller to be an active partner in health care. This reduces the risks associated with misinformed decision making and reduces the delay in seeking advice and direction to the most appropriate health care resource.

A member of the public with a health query can phone the service using a single national telephone number: 0845 46 47. The call is first handled by call-takers, non-nurses, who can then route the call as appropriate. Although people with acute health problems can use NHS Direct, others requiring less urgent services also call. The latter may simply need, for example, the opening times and location of local pharmacies, dental treatment or eye tests. By directing people to the appropriate service, inappropriate attendance at other health service facilities is reduced. If the presenting problem is more serious and illness related, the call is routed by the call-takers to a specially trained nurse who uses computer decision support software to undertake an assessment of the caller's symptoms. This nurse will then take the caller through a series of questions as generated by the decision support software.

## Assessment

The nurse assesses the caller utilising the computer decision support software as a framework to help appraise symptoms and provide advice, treatment and referral options. During the telephone consultation the nurse takes the caller through the assessment presented on the computer screen. The nurse tailors the assessment, which is presented in the form of a number of questions, to the needs of the caller. This allows the caller to be a full participant in the assessment, reducing the risk that the caller does not understand what is being asked of them.

It is important to note that the system software does not dictate to the nurse, but recommends a course of action based on the symptom assessment. The software is not designed to diagnose, but to provide appropriate instruction on the management of presenting symptoms. The assessment process examines the most serious potential reason for presenting symptoms first, and then progresses to less serious causes via a series of logically structured, research based questions embedded within an algorithm. An algorithm, in this context, is the term used for the specific set of assessment questions used in the dialogue with the caller, which are based on the caller's presenting symptoms and relevant variables such as gender and age. On completion of the assessment the caller is either advised who should be contacted and in what time scale, or is provided with comprehensive research based advice to help them manage their symptoms themselves.

## Dispositions

On completion of the assessment the clinical decision support software will recommend a course of action. This is known as the *disposition*. The advice recommended to the caller is a combination of the disposition as given by the software *and* the clinical judgement of the nurse. If the nurse disagrees with the disposition then the assessment is reviewed and a new course of action could be recommended. The system has the capacity to record the consultation as completed using the software (auto document) and so situations in which a disposition recommended by the system is felt to be inappropriate can be reviewed. Furthermore, during the consultation additional information can be entered onto the screen. Once recorded it cannot be deleted, thereby providing a comprehensive risk management tool, through auditable information recording.

The information and advice on the system is regularly reviewed by various National Algorithm Guardian groups who have a responsibility for maintaining and updating the contents of the algorithm. These groups are multi-professional, and form the National Clinical Reference group. Through this mechanism the system is constantly being updated in the light of new clinical evidence and research. This is a major step forward in health care and one that presents a number of advantages. These include access to information on rare health problems and good quality advice on everyday health challenges such as headaches and influenza. Further advice on the latter can be found in the NHS Direct self-help guide entitled *Not Feeling Well* (Banks, 2001). This is a free booklet available to the public from a number of sources including pharmacies and A&E departments. It helps the public to decide when it is safe for them to treat themselves at home.

By providing self-care information, the caller may be enabled to manage the symptoms not only on this occasion, but may also be able to monitor and manage such symptoms on similar occasions in the future. In this sense, NHS Direct can be said to be a health promotion tool. By enabling callers to appropriately manage symptoms, risks associated with inappropriate home treatments are significantly reduced. An example of this is a man in his sixties who used NHS Direct regularly. He stated that 'It is difficult to know how serious something is and I don't like to call the doctor out unnecessarily' (DoH, 2001a p. 13). He subsequently developed chest pain, which was assessed as serious by NHS Direct staff who called an ambulance for him. The opportunity for people with chest pain to receive prompt assessment through NHS Direct will help in meeting the goals set out in the National Service Framework for coronary heart disease (DoH, 2000c).

In addition to the service aspects described above there will be expected levels of symptom sorting, which are closely monitored on an individual, site, network and national basis. This monitoring of where patients are referred to (outcome category), which can include the emergency services, accident and emergency departments (A&E), the GP, or self-care if it is deemed appropriate, is key to the review of individual nurse and system performance. NHS Direct is proactive in seeking feedback from health professionals with regard to the referrals made to ensure that any inappropriate referrals are recognised and form the basis for organisational learning and change. This is achieved by sending evaluation forms to the relevant health care providers within the outcome categories, for example GPs and A&E departments. National performance indicators monitor outputs in terms of clinical safety, accessibility, patient satisfaction and partnership working (DoH, 2001e). Research undertaken at one site in the first year of its operation analysed 56,540 calls and found that self-care (37%) was the commonest outcome category given to callers (Payne & Jessopp, 2001). Of the rest, 28% were advised to see their GP and 6% were referred to A&E.

## The technological infrastructure

There are 22 NHS Direct sites across England and Wales. The sites are divided into four networks, which were derived from the original sites that shared the same software application as the service was being developed. Each site covers a specified geographical area. The current software in use is the Clinical Assessment System, which was introduced in 2000/2001. Call centres vary in size and complement of staff, with each site covering a population size of 1.3 to 4 million people (DoH, 2001a). However the working processes for each are similar. Nurses sit at 'pods' which are workstations with computer terminals. Some have satellite sites, which are smaller call centres within the geographical area covered by the main call centre site. This optimises the ability to meet call volume received by sites and facilitates integration with other sectors of the health service. It also promotes recruitment by enabling nurses to work flexible hours, geographically closer to their own homes.

## *Telephone triage*

Although the pilot sites for NHS Direct in England were introduced in 1997, the utilisation of telephone triage and information has a longer international history. The evidence base for the use of telephone triage is large and it has been used in a number of countries. In Sweden, 20 million calls per year are dealt with by nurses in health centres (Marklund, 1991). Other countries, including Denmark, have utilised national telephone triage systems to facilitate health care access, particularly for remote populations where this can be difficult. The Danish model established mandatory countrywide telephone triage systems although these were staffed, unlike NHS Direct, by general practitioners (Vedsted & Olesen, 1999).

In the United States nurse telephone triage using computer decision support software is well established. The health insurance market is the principal driver behind such systems. The Budget proposal for health by the Clinton administration (NHelp, 1999) provides an insight into how health insurance processes operate in the USA. Some insurers require assessment by a telephone triage nurse before access can be given to health care. In order to gain access the individual must be assessed by the nurse within the call centre and be directed to the appropriate level of care. For example, a caller with diabetes mellitus presenting with recurrent symptoms over a specified timeframe may be directed to a specialist nurse in diabetes who will provide further assessment and advice on disease management. This can reduce the possibility of inappropriate health care intervention and the late presentation of symptoms.

Within the United Kingdom, telephone triage has been in existence for a number of years prior to the introduction of NHS Direct. Most notably A&E departments (Buckles & Carew-McColl, 1991; Jones & Playforth, 2001) and practice nurse assessment of symptoms. Crouch *et al.* (1998) evaluated telephone triage provision from A&E departments and Minor Injury Units, sampling 313 units, with a response rate of 85%. They found that 89% of the sample group placed an emphasis on the importance of telephone triage as part of their role. However, they found that there were limitations on staff training, and a lack of written policy or guidelines on handling calls. The study estimated, based on extrapolated figures for all 313 Minor

Injuries Units and A&E departments across the UK, that some 2 million calls were being dealt with annually. There is no data with regard to whether the details of these calls were recorded. One of the recommendations of the Crouch *et al.* (1998) study was that calls taken by staff in A&E departments could be better dealt with by NHS Direct.

Work undertaken by NHS Direct should be able to relieve the workload of other clinical areas. An example of this is an NHS Direct site triaging the calls of an A&E unit, enabling the department to save two whole time equivalent staff nurse posts per day (Sadler, 2001). This should reduce risk as the calls are dealt with through the NHS Direct system described in this chapter and the staff of A&E are freed up to concentrate on other tasks. Jones and Playforth (2001) found, following the introduction of NHS Direct in the Pontefract (Yorkshire) area, that telephone advice calls handled by the A&E department at Pontefract hospital fell by 72.6%. However, calls made to the hospital switchboard seeking general health advice increased by 315%. This figure was acknowledged to be an overestimate, due to inconsistencies in the way in which calls were recorded, but the rise meant an increase in workload for switchboard staff. It is likely that the number of such calls to hospital switchboards will fall as public awareness of NHS Direct increases.

If a nurse outside of NHS Direct or any other member of the health care team provides information or advice without appropriate training, and calls are not monitored for quality, problems can be envisaged. Furthermore, callers with similar problems may be dealt with differently in different parts of the country or even by different practitioners. Indeed, evidence of differences in advice was found between the early NHS Direct sites by Florin and Rosen (1999). This was probably due to the different software applications being used by those sites. Now that the software for NHS Direct has been standardised this problem no longer exists.

## The NHS Direct software systems

Until September 2000, there had been three computer decision support software systems operating within NHS Direct. These were Centramax, developed by McKesson HBOC, the Telephone Advice System (TAS), developed by The Plain Software Company Limited, and Personal Health Advisor (PHA), also developed by McKesson HBOC. However, such variation within NHS Direct was difficult to justify on financial, logistical or clinical grounds (Florin & Rosen,

1999) and a national procurement programme was initiated to identify and implement a single system for the entire service. By September 2000, the Clinical Assessment System (CAS) had been selected as the standard system. It had been operating for five years in different countries and had dealt with over 7 million calls within a number of clinical contexts, including acute and community care environments (AXA, 2001). The system was chosen via a comprehensive and robust assessment process. This involved selection based on technological and clinical performance, assessed by NHS Direct representatives from nursing, medicine, information technology support and management. It was essential that the system met a number of key criteria including safety, accuracy and consistency, as well as proving credible to staff and callers. It was also essential that the system had defined outcomes, in terms of the expected sorting of symptoms, and was capable of swift adaptation to clinical developments.

The new system was introduced using a phased approach. In order to meet the exacting timetable of introduction, a national training team for NHS Direct was put together. The adoption of a single system was a significant step in reducing the risk associated with the use of multiple assessment systems across the service. The fact that at the time of writing (late 2002) all sites are now using the NHS CAS system should ensure that there will be greater consistency in advice given and more flexibility in terms of dealing with call volume. If a centre is particularly busy, calls can be referred to another centre elsewhere in the country. There is an ongoing evaluation of the CAS software via statistical data, which is collated at individual site level, then passed through to the central project team of NHS Direct. The Department of Health requests these reporting processes, so that service performance can be monitored and managed. This level of performance auditing is unusual within the NHS.

The final report on the first wave sites (Munro *et al.*, 2001), provided some evaluation of the efficacy of the service in terms of patient referral. It concluded that NHS Direct was as safe as any other route to health care, that it had not been unhelpful to other health services, and that it potentially improved the case mix seen by other services. In other words, people were turning up for help at the right point of service, for example A&E or their GP, more frequently. It further concluded that it might have halted the growth of GP out of hours demand. However, the report also noted that with the rapid development of NHS Direct more work was required to assess the effect on changing service demands.

## The utilisation of health services

Clearly NHS Direct has the potential significantly to affect the utilisation of health provision by both individuals and particular social groups. It provides relatively easy and cheap access to health care advice and services, possibly reducing the known gap between socio-economic groups in terms of access. The 0845 46 47 number has a low call charge rate, and with the diversification of access methods including information points, from which free contact can be made, through to the development of nurse-led Walk In Centres (DoH, 1999a), access to health information and treatment should be further enhanced. It is easier and takes less time to make a phone call than to attend a health care facility, of whatever type (Pencheon, 1998).

One of the preliminary findings in the report on NHS Direct (Munro *et al.*, 1998) was that certain sectors of the community were rarely accessing it. These included the elderly, those from ethnic minorities, males aged 20–35 years, those from lower socio-economic groups and those with mental health problems. These groups, perhaps with the exception of the elderly, are known not to use health services effectively. The Payne and Jessopp (2001) study found that the majority of calls concerned children under the age of five.

Further attempts are being made to improve public utilisation of NHS Direct. In terms of the amount of provision, it is still on the increase with the additional services already mentioned coming online. Recent research following an advertising initiative on a national and local level found that spontaneous awareness of NHS Direct was 22% in the context of health care. Prompted awareness of NHS Direct had improved by 10% from October 2000 to 59% in April 2001 (DoH, 2001a). As mentioned earlier, increased public awareness of the service should reduce the number of inappropriate calls made to hospital switchboards (Jones & Playforth, 2000).

The data gathered through NHS Direct could also be a valuable epidemiological tool in the monitoring of specific populations. This may have an impact on the agendas of local health care providers, which have been tasked with maintaining and improving the health of their locality, particularly Primary Care Trusts. This may influence Health Improvement Programmes and work within Health Action Zones (DoH, 1999b), which are areas designated for specific help with regard to health care provision by the government. The full impact of this is yet to be seen, but individual analysis of the calls received is already achievable. This data could be used to help create a health profile for a given geographic area. Through such profiles particular health needs might be identified and appropriate services or education provided.

## Expanding information technology in health care

Work is being undertaken nationally to develop a virtual method of accessing local information, so that all NHS Direct sites can tap into local information as held at site level. If a particular site becomes busy, calls can be passed to another centre, elsewhere in the country, which will have information specific to the location of the caller. This also means that if someone becomes unwell whilst on holiday a call to NHS Direct will be able to provide them with not just a health assessment, but also information about the relevant services in the area they are staying. This is a significant step and one that should ensure that people are given appropriate and accurate information regardless of where, geographically, the call is made from or where the call is dealt with. Once electronic health records are widely available, the potential to enhance communication and the consistency of health advice and treatment through such systems should help to reduce unnecessary harm. For example, concordance with prescribed drug therapies, access to test results, and knowledge about allergies will all be enhanced through an effective electronic health records system.

The capacity of information technology (IT), used in conjunction with telecommunication technology, has allowed NHS Direct not only to formulate links with the sites within the network, but also to implement links with other sectors of the health care system. This has most notably been achieved via the use of the system to develop links with integrated GP out-of-hours cooperatives, where patient assessment details can be transferred to the on-call GP at the press of a button. This may eventually form the basis for integrated care pathways for patients when the NHS Clinical Assessment System, as used in NHS Direct, becomes more widely adopted within the NHS.

Direct links with GP surgeries and Accident and Emergency units already exist in some NHS Direct sites. Evidence from Nottingham and Newcastle has demonstrated that integration into such systems can reduce demand on GP services and reduce referrals to hospital. Further investment will extend such a system to 25 Accident and Emergency sites (DoH, 2001b).

The advantages of the easy transfer of patient details include maximising continuity of care, assuring the accuracy of information and reducing the need for repeated assessment and tests by the various health care providers encountered by the patient. If it is assumed that every health assessment carries a potential risk of harm, accurate health assessment should improve the outcomes of care. The use of IT in the assessment process has been identified as one of the ten key roles for nurses by the Chief Nursing Officer (DoH, 2000a). The emphasis on documentation standards is evident in the clarity of reports and transfer of patient details enabled by such systems, this being reflected within the *Essence of Care* document (DoH, 2001c). This document places an emphasis on accurate, transferable documentation as an expectation of health care delivery, including electronic and multidisciplinary records. Even though problems with data recording for the purposes of research have been noted within NHS Direct (Payne & Jessopp, 2001), it still offers a system through which systematic health and service response data can be collated.

This technological revolution will enhance information exchange and allow those in health care to utilise a more systematic approach to health assessment. However, it could also be argued that the ease with which health care staff can share information about patients and the degree to which individual patients can be tracked might carry risks in terms of confidentiality. Levels of permission and access for staff can be instigated in these computer records systems. In practice, members of the public calling NHS Direct usually accept that their calls will be recorded, as a confidentiality message is heard by the caller at the time of phoning. Information about the call is kept as part of an ongoing computer based record of their contact with the service. Callers can remain anonymous if they wish. This is to reduce any threat that callers may feel and some may have a genuine fear of such surveillance processes, whatever their nature.

## *The role of the nurse in NHS Direct*

The scope of practice presented to nurses within NHS Direct has developed and expanded along with the service. The role is one of a primary nurse, with the potential for the greatest individual case-load ever experienced in nursing. It is also providing new career development opportunities for nurses. Frank Dobson, former Secretary of State for Health, envisaged NHS Direct as contributing to the recruitment and retention of nurses returning to practice, to helping to retain those thinking of leaving practice and those who would have otherwise been unable to maintain a clinical role because of disability (Dobson, 1999).

The experience level required, and pay grades awarded to NHS

Direct staff, has led to some adverse comments from other nurses. It is, however, important to recognise that the nurse is not merely an operator for the computer decision support software, but is required to think critically about clinical decisions and to manage the system appropriately so that callers are safely and comprehensively assessed. The system, although using a robust assessment process in its algorithm base, is only as good as the questions that are asked of the caller. The role of the nurse is to obtain answers to important questions, prompt the provision of relevant further information and symptom history, and interpret this information within the caller's context.

In recognition of the importance of these issues, the processes of induction into NHS Direct have been strengthened, ensuring that nurses are fully trained in the algorithmic software based assessment tool, and also have the ability to utilise the knowledge gained through their clinical experience. Specifically, the training aims to maintain their critical thinking skills, but also to enable them to reflect on their most recent practice so that it does not predetermine, either consciously or subconsciously, the outcome of patient interactions. The objective is that symptoms should be assessed safely and comprehensively, without judgemental or 'knee jerk' reactions. A key advantage of this type of computer software is that it helps to ensure a systematic approach is taken to health assessment.

Following the induction of the practitioner a number of elements and processes exist to reduce unnecessary harm. There is ongoing monitoring of standards of practice, quality reporting mechanisms, support processes, education and training, call monitoring and clinical supervision – all of which fit into a clinical governance framework. This includes a competency framework for the nurses which is being implemented based on an analysis of roles, skill development and the development of effective nurse–patient relationships (DoH, 2001a). All calls are recorded and individual statistics of performance based on a number of variables are drawn from data on the system. These are used to inform the Continuous Quality Improvement (DoH, 2001e) processes of the service, locally and nationally. This information is collated to develop practice and forms a non-punitive approach to problem resolution. In line with the national nursing strategy 'Making a Difference'.

## The clinical governance agenda

It is important that all health care practitioners attempt to reduce the amount of unnecessary harm caused through their interventions.

Such a stance is now enshrined in initiatives such as the National Patient Safety Agency (DoH, 2000b). NHS Direct has the luxury of building clinical governance systems from a new perspective. Clinical governance provides a framework within which to improve and assure the quality of clinical services for patients (DoH, 1999c). It actively takes on board the need for practitioners to understand themselves within the context of practice by promoting the use of clinical supervision to enable a reflective approach to practice. The United Kingdom Central Council position statement on clinical supervision (UKCC, 1996) described it as a process of bringing practitioners and skilled supervisors together to reflect on practice. Clinical supervision aims to identify problems and their potential solutions, to improve practice and to increase the understanding of practice issues encountered during calls. It is actively used in NHS Direct as a method of promoting, safeguarding and enhancing standards of practice.

Through adopting clinical supervision as a real force for change, the service is recognising the need for nurses to be able to address practice concerns with experienced supervisors and in protected time and space, thereby enabling them to arrive at appropriate solutions to presenting problems. An advantage for the practitioner within NHS Direct is that each patient–nurse interaction is recorded and individual calls can therefore be analysed. Call monitoring allows the review of individual nurse performance in terms of the process of telephone triage. It provides effective feedback for the individual nurse on practice performance and can inform the collective practice of the call centre.

The information technology also allows a large amount of statistical analysis in terms of expected sorting in relation to presenting symptoms. This can be used to ensure that the performance of individual nurses and the call centre as a whole is compared with predicted activity, and that inappropriate dispositions do not occur. Examples of such inappropriate dispositions, the outcomes given to the caller, include patients who require medical assistance being advised of self-care measures and patients who require self-care management of symptoms being advised to seek medical intervention. The recording of calls also reduces the potential ambiguity inherent in complaint investigation, and perhaps prompts a more open approach to the reporting of incidents, which team members suspect may cause or may have caused adverse outcomes for patients. This is because there is a 'no blame' culture in which incident investigation is managed quickly and efficiently. The performance monitoring tools, both of the system and the practitioners that operate it, mean that adverse incidents will be evident and relevant data on any such events will be available.

## NHS Direct and the gate-keeping role of GPs

NHS Direct embraces aspects of the gate-keeping role historically associated with GPs in the UK. Members of the public wishing to seek help with their health concerns, other than the very acute for which they might attend A&E, often go to their GP. With the advent of NHS Direct this is changing. There have been mixed reactions to these changes from doctors and GPs in particular, which can be seen in articles and letters in the medical and nursing press (Manocha, 1999; Smith, 1999; Anon, 2000; Duffin, 2000). However, closer examination of the recent government initiatives mentioned in the opening of this chapter suggest that the challenge to GPs is not derived solely from NHS Direct, although it may present the most visible face of change.

The supporters of the system argue that NHS Direct offers an opportunity to provide an acceptable process of graduated access to finite health resources. It satisfies the need for a primary care led NHS, and enables resource rationalisation by acting as a comprehensive sorting mechanism for the appropriate use of health care, while simultaneously meeting the public demand for convenience, quality and access (Pencheon, 1998). There is no evidence that asking people to use nurse-led access to health care will result in inappropriate increased demand (Brown & Armstrong, 1995; Pencheon, 1998). Furthermore, Lattimer *et al.* (1998) provided evidence that the outcome of nurse-led triage using support software resulted in no adverse effects. In reality there are extensive examples of collaborative working between medical colleagues and NHS Direct, particularly in terms of out-of-hours GP work being triaged by NHS Direct. Prior to the implementation of NHS Direct, many GP cooperatives used nursing expertise to provide triage for providing prioritisation and advice for out-of-hours callers. The introduction of the Exemplar Programme (DoH, 2001d) aims to establish standards of practice for out-of-hours performance by NHS Direct and GPs.

## The future

Before considering future developments it is important to acknowledge that the combination of practitioner skills aided by computer support in health assessment is not new. As already mentioned, such systems have been used in other countries for some time. Computers have also been used in the UK to aid the diagnostic process. Work by de Dombal (1991) describes the introduction and use of computer decision support software in aiding the diagnosis of abdominal pain. The software was used on over 30,000 cases seen in more than ten hospitals over a period of 13 years. The computer compared the symptom presentation pattern of the patient with the information held on a database, and then made a diagnostic recommendation. The initial history, examination and investigations were made and requested by the clinician and the final decision about diagnosis remained with the clinician. The significance of the work by de Dombal is that it demonstrated that such systems were feasible for use in clinical practice when used as an adjunctive tool. The research, undertaken in the early 1980s, concluded that the system improved diagnostic accuracy and reduced unnecessary investigations, thereby cutting cost and the risks, pain and inconvenience associated with additional invasive tests and unnecessary surgery. However, they were not to be used widely in practice. It is known that levels of unnecessary or inappropriate surgery remain high (Sharpe & Faden, 1998), as described in Chapter 2.

NHS Direct is a clear (although for some a controversial) example of the value of information technology in improving communication and consistency within health care. The balance that it embraces, practitioner experience and computer software based guidance to decision making, is a model that could be repeated in a multitude of health care contexts. This combination may well make a valuable contribution to the reduction of unnecessary harm in health care. The NHS is investing £200 million in modernising IT systems and an extra £250 million will be invested in 2003/2004. Further innovations include electronic appointment booking, the introduction of electronic patient records by 2005 (DoH, 2002), electronic prescribing of medicines by 2004, and facilities for telemedicine by 2005 (DoH, 2000a). There is then the possibility that this opportunity will be taken and we may see IT used more effectively in the attempt to reduce unnecessary harm.

Web based telephone technology could allow decision support software systems to be carried by primary care practitioners in the community to assist them in assessing the individuals they visit. The outcome of the assessment could then be used as the basis for care implementation. The information could then be downloaded to a central electronic patient record thus enhancing continuity of care. The central development team of NHS Direct is enhancing the use of web based technology as a method for undertaking symptom assessment for callers who choose this medium of communication. Some people will find access online easier than using a telephone and this method carries advantages for those with a hearing impairment. The NHS Direct web site already receives approximately 4.6 million hits per month (DoH, 2001a).

It is likely that in the medium term it will become common for people to be assessed with reference to an IT based system. Computers will not and cannot replace all aspects of the judgement and adaptability of practitioners, but they can supplement and enhance that process. For example, we may see information technology and the relevant algorithms utilised in areas as diverse as the paramedic attending a road traffic accident through to community psychiatric nurses assessing a person with symptoms of depression and anxiety. If we desire evidence based practice, we need access to that evidence, and even using the technology readily available today, it is possible to provide this to practitioners wherever they are, be it hospital or community.

## *Conclusion*

The nature and organisation of health care in any society is representative of the character of the society that it operates within. Across the globe people continue to embrace technology in its various guises, and communication technology in particular. Such changes are now reflected in the UK with the introduction of NHS Direct, which is already the largest provider of telephone accessed health advice in the world (DoH, 2001a). Such innovation had been limited within the NHS prior to the inception of NHS Direct. It marks a radical rethinking in that it challenges the historical reliance of the public upon initial face to face consultation when they have health concerns. Furthermore, if the public accesses health care staff and services more appropriately, this will free time and resources for face to face contact where this is appropriate.

There are limits to what can be achieved through information giving and the remote assessment of symptoms, yet NHS Direct is representative of the opportunities inherent in the effective use of IT in health care. The government goals referred to in this chapter show that services within the NHS will continue to be integrated through IT, breaking many of the barriers to effective communication currently in place. It is envisaged that the gate-keeping role traditionally held by general practitioners will be refocused as the nature of the demand for that service will shift. NHS Direct will enable the general public by increasing their health related knowledge, providing accurate and reliable health assessment and if necessary direct them to places where they can obtain help and treatment. It will, along with the other innovations mentioned here, reduce the clinical risk to patients by strategic use of evidence based information technology ensuring a consistent approach to care and treatment within a robust clinical governance framework.

**Reducing harm in health care: lessons from NHS Direct**

| |
|---|
| i. The use of computer decision support software can enhance assessment and referral processes in health care reducing the risk of unnecessary harm occurring. |
| ii. Nurses can use information technology to improve the health of the public they work with. |
| iii. Information technology can improve public access to health related information. |
| iv. Clinical governance can be facilitated through the use of appropriate information technology. |
| v. Computerised systems could be used more widely to enhance acute health assessment and collate health related data. |

## References

Anon (2000) NHS Direct. *British Medical Journal.* **321**, 446.

AXA (2001). *AXA Assistance CAS. NHS Nurse Information, Pre-Training Workbook.* AXA, Leatherhead.

Banks, I. (2001) *The NHS Direct Self Help Guide. Not Feeling Well.* Department of Health, London.

Brown, A. & Armstrong, D. (1995) Telephone consultation in general practice: an additional or alternative service? *British Journal of General Practice.* **45**, 673–675.

Buckles, E. & Carew-McColl, M. (1991) Triage by telephone. *Nursing Times.* **87**, (6) 26–28.

Campbell, H., Hotchkiss, R., Bradshaw. N. & Porteous. M. (1998) Integrated care pathways. *British Medical Journal.* **316** (7125), 133–137.

Crouch, R., Dale, J., Visaradia, B. & Higton, C. (1998) Provision of telephone advice from Accident and Emergency departments. A national survey. *Journal of Accident and Emergency Medicine.* **16**, 112–113.

de Dombal, F. T. (1991) Computer-aided diagnosis of acute abdominal pain: the British experience. In: *Professional Judgement: A reader in clinical decision making* (eds J. Downie & A. Elstein), pp. 190–199. Cambridge University Press, Cambridge.

DoH (1997) *The New NHS, Modern and Dependable.* Department of Health, London.

DoH (1998) *A First Class Service – Quality in the New NHS.* HSC 1999/116. Department of Health, London.

DoH (1999a) *NHS Primary Care Walk in Centres.* Department of Health, London.

DoH (1999b) *Saving Lives – Our Healthier Nation.* Department of Health, London.

DoH (1999c) *Clinical Governance in the New NHS.* Health Service Circular HSC 1999/065. Department of Health, London.

DoH (2000a) *The NHS Plan. A plan for investment. A plan for reform.* Department of Health, London.

DoH (2000b) *An Organisation with a Memory. Report of an expert group on learning from adverse events in the NHS chaired by the Chief Medical Officer.* The Stationery Office, London.

DoH (2000c) *National Service Framework for Coronary Heart Disease.* Department of Health, London.

DoH (2001a) *NHS Direct. A new gateway to healthcare.* Department of Health, London.

DoH (2001b) *Reforming Emergency Care.* Department of Health, London.

DoH (2001c) *Essence of Care. Patient focused benchmarking for healthcare practitioners.* Department of Health, London.

DoH (2001d) *Raising Standards for Patients. New partnerships in out of hours care. An independent review of out of hours services in England.* Department of Health, London.

DoH (2001e) *NHS Direct. The new performance framework: improving quality.* Consultation paper, December. Department of Health, London.

DoH (2002) *Learning from Bristol: The Department of Health's response to the Report of the Public Inquiry into children's heart surgery at the Bristol Royal infirmary 1984–1995.* The Stationery Office, London.

Dobson, F. (1999) A direct hit. *Nursing Times.* **95** (33), 32.

Duffin, C. (2000) Ringing the changes. *Nursing Standard.* **15** (12), 14–15.

Florin, D. & Rosen, R. (1999) Evaluating NHS Direct. *British Medical Journal.* **319** (7201) 5–6.

Jones, J. & Playforth, M. J. (2001) The effect of the introduction of NHS Direct on requests for telephone advice from an accident and emergency department. *Emergency Medicine Journal.* **18**, 300–301.

Latimer, V., George, S., Thompson, F., Mullee, M. & Turnbull, J. (1998) Safety and effectiveness of nurse telephone consultation in out of hours primary care: randomised control trial. *British Medical Journal.* **317**, 1054–1059.

Manocha, R. (1999) New threat to GPs' role as gatekeepers. *General Practitioner.* **12** (March), 1.

Marklund, B. (1991) How well do nurse-run telephone consultations in surgery agree? Experience in Swedish primary healthcare. *British Journal of General Practice.* **41**, 462–465.

McLellan, N. (1999) NHS Direct: here and now. *Archives of Childhood Diseases.* **81**, 376–379.

Munro, J., Nicholl, J., O'Caithan, A. & Knowles, E. (1998) *Evaluation of NHS Direct First Wave Sites. First Interim Report to the Department of Health.* Sheffield Medical Care Research Unit, University of Sheffield.

Munro, J., Nicholl, J., O'Caithan, A., Knowles, E. & Morgan, A. (2001) *Evaluation of NHS Direct First Wave Sites. Final Report of the Phase 1 Research.* Sheffield Medical Care Research Unit, University of Sheffield.

NHelp (1999) *President Clinton's proposed budget on health.* Available from http:nhelp.org

Payne, F. & Jessopp, L. (2001) NHS Direct: review of activity data for the first year of operation at one site. *Journal of Public Health Medicine.* **23**, 155–158.

Pencheon, D. (1998) NHS Direct: managing demand. *British Medical Journal.* **316**, 215–216.

Sadler, M. (2001) Dial M for ... Medical Advice. *Health Service Journal.* **111** (5756), 24–26.

Sharpe, V. A. & Faden, A. I. (1998) *Medical Harm: Historical, conceptual, ethical dimensions of iatrogenic illness.* Cambridge University Press, Cambridge.

Smith, N. (1999) GP's welcome radical new out-of-hours plan. *General Practitioner.* **12** (March), 2.

UKCC (1996) *The UKCC Position Statement on Clinical Supervision.* United Kingdom Central Council for Nursing, Midwifery & Health Visiting, London.

Vedsted, P. & Olesen, F. (1999) Effect of a reorganised after-hours service on frequent attenders. *Family Medicine.* **31**, 270–275.

# 12. *Avoiding Harm in Medical Care – A Doctor's Perspective*

## *Donald Richardson*

> All professions are conspiracies against the laity.
> George Bernard Shaw, 1911

### *Introduction*

Doctors have always harmed some of those they treat, and they always will. The reasons range from the inevitable to the indefensible. It is unavoidable that much of medical practice is an uncertain business and that disease processes are not fully understood. It is also unavoidable that individuals show biological variations and are different in intelligence, psychology and emotions. All of these factors are relevant to how an individual will respond to what is meant to be a healing process of body, mind or both.

Doctors are human beings and are therefore prone to error. Factors external and internal to the doctor affect the susceptibility to error in varying circumstances. Like everyone else, doctors may also be sad, mad or bad. These human factors may have serious outcomes in harm to those who put their trust in healers. This chapter expands on these ideas and their effects on practice.

### *Health and disease*

There is a fundamental difference between health, which is a personal and societal construct, and health care, which is the personal response of an individual health care professional to someone who has come seeking to be rid of their personal 'dis-ease'. The delivery of health care may be within a commercial, charitable or state provided infrastructure but the relationship of the professional to the patient is intense, personal, emotional, often dependent and open to exploitation on both sides. This is why there is scope for harm and an ethical duty to avoid it.

The norms of 'health' are arbitrary. We all decide for ourselves what to adopt amongst the huge range of 'ideals' presented to us by the state, by advertisers, by sportspeople, by beauticians, by bodybuilders, and by a host of others. What do we hope to achieve? It may be physical prowess, it may be longevity, it may be a beautiful body size and image, it may be lots of things. But many of us simply do not care that smoking and a fatty diet will make our lives shorter than the average.

This is where the state comes in, essentially so on an environmental basis and often so on an economic basis. Once a society has clean water and adequate food, warmth and shelter and there is sufficient economic activity to make these basic essentials attainable by most of the population, the health stance of the state becomes economic. Its goal is primarily to reduce death occurring earlier than the average, and to avoid excessive sickness absence from work. There will always be a dominant cause of death. Societies always have and always will vary in what is regarded, often irrationally, as an acceptable distribution of mortality and morbidity.

Many developed countries, especially those of a Judaeo-Christian moral inheritance, have evolved a greater altruism and are prepared to devote a substantial proportion of the state's wealth to health care, often through redistributive taxation processes. This meets the moral obligation of a society to support its less able citizens. It is also an attempt to generalise and accommodate all the personal decisions about 'dis-ease' which I describe above. This is an impossible task (Porter, 1997). The result of this relatively easy general availability of good quality health advice and care is an older but overall less fit society. In the UK and similar societies we all spend much longer 'unwell' before we die than used to be the case. The consequence is that the altruism of easily available health care has to be modified by setting criteria of 'health', limiting what can be provided by the state. There seems to be no limit to the resources that could be expended on sustaining the longer 'unwell' life. The dilemma is that our choices for ourselves and our loved ones conflict directly with the 'greatest benefit' choices the state (which is all of us acting collectively) has to make (DoH, 1998a & b).

The potential for state sponsored 'harm' arising from these processes is outside the scope of this chapter, which concentrates on personal doctor-caused harm in the treatment of disease, but underlies the reality of daily health care practice in the UK and similar societies. It controls what we are to decide is, in scientific terms, a disease and how it should be treated. Invasion by an infecting agent may be easy to identify as disease, although even here there can be discussion about the 'normal' level of the presence of parasites or of some bacteria. Everyone may have some but in excess, or in others, there may be serious disease consequences. Much more difficult to define are the large number of non-infectious, but nevertheless seriously disabling conditions which are due to variations in 'normal' body function. All body functions and characteristics show the normal bell-shaped distribution curve of all biological variables. The cut off points for abnormality, whether high or low, are generally arbitrary, hence the cliché that 'the only healthy person is the one who has not been fully investigated yet'.

The practical consequence is the maxim that it is usually better to treat the patient and not the investigations. Unfortunately, there are common conditions, such as hypertension, where this is not so. Above average blood pressure takes many years to produce the irreversible changes that cause symptoms and premature death. Treating apparently healthy people raises dilemmas, especially if the treatment is not free of inconvenience or risk, in order to avoid much greater future risk. Even more controversial is deciding what is to be regarded as 'normal' in the degenerative 'wearing out' processes associated with increasing age. There is huge individual variation in incidence and severity. Most treatment is relief not cure. As with all treatment, the patient will decide what is done, but who decides what to offer and with what chance of benefit and at what cost?

It is the function of public health doctors and nurses to understand and explain these dilemmas. In our irrational quest for a risk-free society, where everything adverse is someone's fault and should never have happened, it is hard to get public acceptance of possible harm to a tiny number of individuals for the benefit of everyone else. The criteria for the acceptance of immunisation and screening programmes encapsulate these problems (Health Departments of the United Kingdom, 1998).

## Health care delivery

It is unusual for any individual not to be aware at all times of some bodily function that is amiss, possibly in a very trivial way. Health care begins when we decide that the triviality barrier has been broken and we seek a consultation with a suitable professional.

'The [study of the] history of medicine teaches the student to use their imagination, their spirit of enquiry and to try to accept the humility of ignorance. These are virtues for which doctors are not well known.'

Ford, 2001 p. 13

In many fields of medical practice it is unusual to know exactly everything that is wrong with the person seeking help. Treatment recommendations are made on a balance of probabilities. It follows that the recommendations will sometimes be wrong, resulting in harm, because the improbable, but not impossible, has happened. Even when there is substantial certainty and the treatment recommendation is correct, the outcome may be harm. The physician knows the effect of a particular drug or other treatment on most people. The current patient may be an exception to the norm for physiological or psychological reasons. The surgeon may be very familiar with the anatomy usually to be found in a particular situation but the current patient may be different, leading to operative difficulties and harm. An individual may react in unexpected ways to psychotherapy. Every new treatment or prescription and every surgical operation is, to a degree, an experiment. Experiments do not always turn out as expected.

The consultation process has several stages. The patient's problem must be clarified by questioning. Examination and testing will bring more evidence. The doctor will reach a reasoned conclusion, explain it to the patient and discuss how the problem may best be tackled. The patient decides what is acceptable and then both doctor and patient discuss how far that agreed need is achievable with the facilities and resources available in the circumstances in which they are.

Doctors may be prejudiced and anxious patients may not be rational, so disrupting this orderly process. 'I'll leave it to you, doctor' may encourage a paternalistic vainglory (Williamson, 1992). 'I saw this treatment on the web' may lead to a chase after a will-o'-the-wisp idea dressed up as a scientific hypothesis which, in fact, has no more validity than the 'humours' and 'bile' of the ancients (Porter, 1997).

What can be done in remote circumstances will differ from what can be done in a modern city centre. Where medical care is a market-place commodity, the patient's means may limit what can be done.

We are all vulnerable to the insidious manipulation of the snake-oil salesman and his present-day successors. We chase any idea

239

which purports to offer relief where none has been previously found or, for some conditions, where none exists. Harm from treatment may result and is, to a degree, self-inflicted. We all at first clutch at straws for our loved ones or for ourselves. Doctors must try to bring balance and, in particular, explain the strength of the evidence which suggests that benefit may be expected from a particular course of action. Professionals must not confuse science, individual experience, anecdote, faith and hope. All may be legitimate but patient and professional must know what they are doing and why. Uncontrolled or concealed reliance on human suggestibility, which is enormous, and the placebo effect, which is universal, is unprofessional (Porter, 1997). Autonomous individuals must not, overtly or covertly, be denied the right to decide the limits of the treatment which they are willing to accept. An informed 'enough is enough' decision must be respected if professionals, however well intentioned, are to avoid causing much harm and distress.

## Health and health care advice

There are now many sources of advice on health and health care, from the state provided NHS Direct (see Chapter 11), through learned bodies, to pressure groups and commercial organisations, not all of which are disinterested in selling either insurance or 'health' products. There is a plethora of leaflets, booklets and health care guides ranging from those available free from doctor or pharmacy to large volumes which will make a big hole in a book-buying budget. Careful usage and reading can help many people to understand the state's 'health' initiatives and to decide whether, how and when they should seek professional advice. But there is no substitute for professional face-to-face personalised advice directed to achieving greatest benefit at least risk.

Each of us will define why and when we will seek advice and decide for ourselves whether we like and will accept that advice. The search for a 'cure' is often chimerical. All injuries leave traces, even if only a minor skin scar. Most other treatment, surgical or medical, simply removes the offending part, suppresses or counteracts the offending function, or artificially replaces, perhaps for the rest of life, the destroyed process. Doctors must accept patients' wishes but must not carry out second best procedures if the harm they may bring could be avoided, but doctor and patient may have to accept second best if it is forced upon them by circumstances.

## Iatrogenic harm in history

From earliest recorded times, societies have tried to protect their citizens from harm from healers, whether from ignorance or exploitation. The written records remaining of the Mesopotamian civilisations from the seventh century BC onwards contain much guidance for physicians on the best practice of the day. By about 1600 BC, the great king Hammurabi laid down clinical and administrative instructions for physicians. Success in treatment, especially of a lord, was well rewarded. Amputating the physician's hand punished failure. Death of a treated slave required the healer to become that slave. Such harsh 'reward by results' regimes may have reduced harm, but by Hippocratic times, around 400 BC, Greek scientific method of observation, experiment and conclusion was beginning to be developed under the most quoted Hippocratic aphorism, rendered into Latin later as 'primum non nocere' – first, do no harm (Porter, 1997).

That is still the underlying philosophy of treatment today. The challenge is to achieve 'no harm' against the background described above.

## Medical education and training

The process has to begin with the choosing of future doctors. Since the late 1950s the UK has trained as doctors a substantial proportion of the highest achievers in school. The hope is that in 10 to 15 years from leaving school, these young people will be empathetic adults, confident in the technical skills they have acquired for their chosen speciality, good listeners, good communicators, constantly self-critical, constantly learning, supportive of colleagues who find the challenge too great and always knowing where the line must be drawn to avoid harm to the public. To achieve these ends they must be shown how to live with uncertainty. They must be able to manage personal failure. They will fail sometimes, not necessarily culpably, but someone who has put their trust in them will have suffered, possibly died. They must learn how to learn from the experience, and from the experiences of others, so that they can come confidently to assess and manage the risky environment in which they work. This training will deliver confidence in personal abilities and knowledge of personal limitations (GMC, 2001a).

Training must include the management of ignorance. Much is understood about normal bodily function, from the mechanics of skeletal movement to the cell biology of individual organs. Much is known of the causation of disease but there remain badly understood areas. Not enough is known about the detailed function of some parts of the body, like the brain. A complete picture of all the effects of many disease conditions has not yet been achieved. Many causations are labelled 'not known' or 'poorly understood'. Also frequently not fully understood is the detailed interaction of body and mind which can profoundly affect both disease and treatment in any individual. Many past practices, from bleeding, cupping and purging, through heroic surgery for cancer, most tonsillectomies and six weeks in bed for heart attacks have all been shown to be wrong, harmful or a waste of time (Porter, 1997).

Many current treatments are unproven, thought unnecessary, too demanding on patients, too costly in money, time or people to be justifiable, too trivial or just the fad of the moment. Some will follow into oblivion what has gone before. Doctors must know how to recognise these factors, assess the criteria against which judgements have been made and change what they do accordingly.

In training, doctors must be resigned to grasping, understanding, retaining and knowing how to access the ever-increasing body of current knowledge. They must acquire and constantly hone by practice the technical skills needed to avoid harm. They must be able through constant practice to rely on their history taking skills being complete, thorough and consistently reproducible so that pressures of patient numbers against available time do not compromise standards. Cutting corners is an avoidable cause of harm. Checklists, protocols and computer driven algorithm systems can all help, but will not improve quality if they are used in an automatic 'one size fits all' way. Health care delivery is above all about what is appropriate for that individual patient. General practitioners in training are constantly reminded that the question they are seeking to answer is 'Why is *this* patient, seeing *me*, presenting *these symptoms*, in *this way, today*?' Assessment and diagnosis, or provisional diagnosis, is not complete until all these questions have been answered and a plan of action formulated in physical, psychological and social terms, and agreed with the patient (Taylor, 1954; Porter, 1997).

The language used in reaching this agreement with the patient can also be a source of harm. Many patients, especially the mentally ill, see diagnoses simply as labels with stereotyping value judgements attached to them. Incautious references, especially to prognosis, can be counter-productive in that they can become a barrier to further explanation and discussion.

## Sustaining autonomy and confidence

Constant teaching, constant guidance from colleagues and from the literature and a reflective approach to all they do will enhance the skill and confidence needed for doctors to take autonomous decisions which are as correct as they can be. Teamwork with many colleagues is usual today in many types of practice but it is still usually a doctor who will take the ultimate decision about what is to be advised to the patient. As a consequence, the doctor will carry the ultimate professional responsibility for that decision.

It is less easy to manage those who do not recognise that the limits of their personal knowledge and skills is a source of harm to patients. 'You don't know what you don't know' and therefore can harm patients. In this situation, the team should come into its own in providing a moderating influence to rash or wrong decisions, support after an adverse event or, if necessary, a way into retraining for the failing doctor. In initial training, doctors must be taught how teams work and how to work in a team.

## Professional requirements

Since the beginning of the twentieth century most countries have required that anyone aspiring to the social cachet of medical doctor must have minimum standards of competency. Statutory bodies have been created to set the standards and oversee their attainment. In the UK the General Medical Council (GMC) oversees the undergraduate curriculum and the compliance of medical schools in delivering it. It has recently revised its basic policy document *Tomorrow's Doctors* (GMC, 2001a) to ensure that new medical graduates have the grounding to develop the characteristics described above. The GMC also maintains a register of those reaching the required standard, whether educated in the UK or abroad. It also tries to make sure that doctors who abuse the trust of the public are either helped to reform or stopped from being registered medical practitioners. Doctors must minimise the potential for harm in their practices by adherence to the sets of guidelines which the GMC produces in order to protect the public (GMC, 2001b).

There have been events in recent times in the UK where long-standing poor standards of practice by individuals, or within whole hospital departments, have come to light. Government and public have therefore questioned the ability of the GMC to provide adequate protection from poor and dangerous practice. Serious criminal activity has also gone undetected (CHI, 2001; Herbert, 2001). Reform is in progress and UK legislation will follow.

Since the late 1990s the GMC has placed an explicit duty on doctors to do something about colleagues whose standards cause concern because of actual or potential patient harm (GMC, 1997). The possible causes are many. The burned out doctor, over-whelmed by pressures applied to them but unable or unwilling to see the falling standards which have resulted. The idle doctor, perhaps misplaced in the career to begin with, totally unmotivated to keep up with changing methods and ideas and uncaring of the consequences. The doctor stressed through personal matters unre-lated directly to work, but preoccupied and therefore allowing standards to slip. Some of these individuals will take to drink or drugs. The benevolent 'carrying' of such doctors by colleagues cannot be accepted if patients are to be protected from harm. Some doctors may be physically or mentally ill but determined to 'carry on' for their patients when they should no longer do so. They must be stopped. A very few doctors are bad, calculatedly exploiting for financial reasons the trust placed in them or seeking to gratify sexual desires or extreme personality traits, such as enjoyment of killing people. Where such a doctor is otherwise good at the job and respected, identification can be very difficult and removal from practice long delayed (Herbert, 2001).

Such identification of failure may be very difficult even for pro-fessional colleagues. The consulting room is often a very private place with, after the end of training, no monitoring by others of what takes place inside it. Even in specialist hospital practice, involving many others besides doctors, 'whistleblowers' have not been welcomed and have, until recently, had no formal protection (NHS Executive, 1999a). A number of people may know a little to the disadvantage of an individual practitioner but coordination of this information, and acting upon it appropriately, while main-taining necessary confidentiality, is extremely difficult to do.

## Health care delivery systems

The health care delivery system within which the doctor works is crucial to enabling high standards of professional performance that cause as little harm as possible. In the UK, few people seek health care as a marketplace commodity. Such a doctor and patient relationship is comparatively easy to manage, although, as with any 'piecework' system of payment, it can lead to over-investigation and overtreatment by unscrupulous practitioners. It was shown many years ago that in populations of similar size in apparently socially identical parts of the United States, the number of hysterectomies carried out related only to the number of gynaecologists in practice and not to the demography or social characteristics of the population.

It is more difficult to manage the doctor–patient relationship where the state provides the infrastructure for the delivery of professional work. Resource constraints can impinge on standards to the extent of causing harm which is not of the doctor's making. The doctor has a duty to make sure that those responsible for resource allocation understand the consequences if there are clinical shortcomings in existing or proposed resource provision. Ultimately a doctor has a responsibility to the public, as patients, and to the registration body, to make known any potential for harm (BMJ, 1993).

## Quality in the UK National Health Service

Almost all the practising doctors in the UK work within the National Health Service (NHS). Since 1997 the corporate structure of the service has made much more explicit the need for a working environment dedicated to quality, and therefore to the avoidance of risk and harm to patients. Every chief executive of every NHS body has a personal accountability for the quality of what that body does. The concept of clinical governance (NHS Executive, 1999b) provides an administrative infrastructure and material support for the organisation to ensure that its clinical systems are risk assessed and managed and allows health professionals, including doctors, to examine critically every aspect of their work. An important part of this process is to recognise the inherent risks in whatever is being undertaken and take all possible steps to control and minimise those risks both in people and in systems in order to reduce potential and actual patient harm.

The essence is to choose the right people, train them properly for the job, give them the right tools to do it with and train them in correct use, set clinical standards against relevant criteria, establish protocols and systems for safe working, monitor and audit the achievement of the standards and the application of the protocols, have a 'no blame' culture for the recognition, reporting and investigation of adverse events, including near misses, learn from complaints, support everyone in career-long learning and career development and produce improvement through research and development activities. The items in this list are time consuming to carry out and need financial and administrative support. Where everyone is co-operating and clinical governance is working well, the NHS can already demonstrate improvement in the quality of practice by doctors and nurses and, therefore, reduction in harm and risks of harm for patients. (NHS Executive, 1999b; van Zwanenberg & Harrison, 2000).

## UK *national quality structures*

Supporting these activities are national bodies. In England and Wales these are the National Institute for Clinical Excellence (NICE), the Commission for Health Improvement (CHI), The National Clinical Assessment Authority (NCAA), and the National Patient Safety Agency (NPSA). Similar bodies are to be created in Scotland and Northern Ireland. There is also to be a UK-wide Council for the Regulation of Healthcare Professionals (CRHP) (DoH, 2001).

NICE assists in the avoidance of harm through considering in detail the effects of various treatments and drugs, especially in fields where differing clinical views exist or where new treatments become available. It aims to produce guidance on the best and most cost-effective treatments. Its task is especially difficult in the drugs field. Most treatments have a balance of benefit and harm. No medication is totally free of unwanted harmful side effects. These may be quite minor in most people, although possibly serious for some individuals. Some treatments always cause serious side effects, such as some chemotherapy agents for malignant disease. The balance of benefit to harm is always one for the patient to decide but it is essential that professionals know and give clearly to patients the information needed to reach a decision on what they will find personally acceptable.

Control of drug development prior to marketing is much more stringent than was the case in the past but rare harmful effects may not become apparent in initial trials. A national reporting system is in place on which continued use decisions can be made. Doctors must understand and use these systems to contribute to recognition of harm and avoid it in their practice. These systems of the UK Medicines Control Agency can be expanded to allow recognition of problems arising from nurse prescribing as the authorised formulary is expanded.

A major difficulty is controlling safety in drug treatment in children, where potential risk in conventional controlled drug trials may be ethically unacceptable, and in the treatment of rare diseases, where there may not be sufficient numbers to justify the enormous cost of safe development by drug companies of new treatments, or to provide for statistically valid and ethically acceptable trials. In these circumstances, there is no substitute for careful judgement and experience based on trial and error development, but at inevitably greater risk for the patient.

Some treatments bring benefits that are short-lived, minor or apparent only in a small minority of patients. NICE's recommendations about some of these treatments have provoked controversy with some patient groups who seek for their members some relief, however small, from progressive disease.

CHI has a continuous monitoring role of the effectiveness, including avoidance of harm, of the services offered by NHS bodies, including general practices. If a serious event has occurred it may be asked to assess the reasons and advise on future avoidance.

The NCAA will help to identify, assist, support and retrain doctors whose clinical performance standards give their employers or their colleagues cause for concern. It will be backed up by clearer processes for what is given the pejorative name of 'whistleblowing', but which is properly part of a health professional's duty of care to patients (DoH, 2000a).

The NPSA will put in place systems for central reporting from all of the NHS and from research bodies of all events giving rise to actual or potential patient harm, including near misses, and derive recommendations for changes of practice from those reports. Its initial targets include reduction or elimination of already identified failures which are indefensible, such as incorrect intrathecal injections (DoH, 2000b). The CRHP will oversee the activities of the various professional registration bodies to ensure that their primary focus is always on the needs of patients rather than of the professionals (NHS, 2001a).

The medical defence societies have undertaken much work on the assessment and avoidance of medical risk, based on matters that have given rise to complaint or litigation against doctors, and advise their members on techniques for the avoidance of patient harm (MDU, 2000). The Clinical Negligence Scheme for Trusts performs a similar service for NHS Trusts in ensuring that systems are in place to avoid well-known risks and that they are adhered to.

## Quality in practice

There is thus no shortage of knowledge about the causes and likelihood of patient harm in any field of practice and no shortage of practical support and advice on how to assess and avoid risk.

It is up to doctors to obtain and keep current that knowledge and apply all the time in their practice the appropriate and necessary risk assessment and harm avoidance techniques. Doctors are now to be tested on how well they do that. The NHS is to appraise annually the performance of all its doctors. The GMC will require all doctors to be re-accredited in their chosen field of work, at regular intervals. Doctors will be required to keep records of their practice and activities which are relevant to quality performance. Where deficiencies are identified, support and retraining will be available in both mechanisms to try to improve work quality. Some doctors may need to be helped to accept physical or psychological treatment for themselves (NHS, 2001a; 2001b).

Serious failure will be dealt with within the NHS through disciplinary procedures and by the GMC by prevention of practice, limitation of practice or, where irredeemable features are present, by permanent removal from the Register. This does not necessarily prevent work in the health field. NHS employment is not possible, and other employment unlikely, but it is perfectly lawful for anyone to offer the public treatment of any sort provided there is no pretence to be a registered medical practitioner.

No doctor who practises correctly and conscientiously has anything to fear from these processes nor, more to the point, have their patients, but there are barriers to achieving quality in current NHS practice in too many places in the UK. Many doctors find themselves constantly pressed by the volume of work presenting to them. Working continuously under a sense of pressure is demoralising and demotivating. There develops a constant feeling of not doing things as well or as thoroughly as is needed. Good training and increasing experience will ensure that patient risk is minimised, but it is not easy to maintain this and eventually it will prove impossible to maintain because of personal burn out. Doctors retire early to escape from these pressures.

In some fields there are not enough trained people to do the work which presents. Solving this is a much longer-term problem. It takes ten to fifteen years to train doctors in any field to be safely and confidently autonomous. Some specialities are of less appeal than others, sometimes because of their intrinsic nature and sometimes because of the current organisational structure within which the particular type of care is delivered. The potential for patient harm is increased where services are short of necessary expertise and those with the expertise have always to run against an increasing workload. There is often no material recognition or even acknowledgement of efforts to continue offering the best possible care in the circumstances. There is also a shortage of other health care skills, besides those of doctors, hindering the effective working of teams.

Some places have a poor infrastructure of buildings, equipment, staff availability and management support. Risk of patient harm is increased where organisation is not conducive or directed to avoiding harm. Some potential risks of harm are well known and foreseeable. Protocols to avoid such things as the wrong doses of drugs, especially in children, the removal of wrong limbs or the incorrect route of drug giving are well known, but errors still occur. System and equipment design to avoid harm through foreseeable human error needs constant refinement, constant review of usage methods, rapid appreciation and adoption of new ideas to minimise harm and thorough audit of current practice leading to positive change where needed (Williamson, 1992).

## Doctors and their conduct

Most patients are not harmed. Most doctors practise well and carefully most of the time in a way that benefits the patient. Most doctors are empathetic, well adjusted, caring, mature individuals anxious to apply their skills in a way which does not harm their patients and which gives to the doctor the sustaining self-esteem of recognising a good job done well. There are ways to assist the achievement of these desirable goals and to assist the self-recognition of non-achievement before it becomes a habitual way of life and practice that, sooner or later, will lead to patient harm.

The first need for all doctors is to ingrain into themselves a determination never to betray the trust which people place in them and their skills. This involves clarity of underlying objectives and an adherence to those requirements of the profession which explicitly include providing a quality service to the public (GMC, 2001b). This is commonly expressed as adding life to years, not just years to life. The life in question is not the doctor's; it is the patient's. We all decide how we wish to live our lives and how much notice we will take of advice which we may be given about healthy living or the treatment of ill health. At a wider social level we decide through our political choices what distribution of the inevitable 100% mortality fits with our current view of an acceptable society. We all accept a degree of risk or likelihood of harm to ourselves and our longevity through our choices for traffic laws, housing standards, industrial pollution, clean water and food and many other things (DoH,

1998a). For many of us this acceptance is implicit rather than explicit, or often not thought about at all, but it forms the background to the level of risk we will accept for ourselves in the health and health care advice which we take. It follows that doctors must know the potential risks of the advice being given, must know the demonstrated actual risks from all sources of what is proposed and must be full and honest in explaining to the patient the nature of potential harm.

Doctors must therefore be good communicators, good at listening to people and good at assessing the level of understanding achieved or achievable with particular individuals. Not only must they be good at communicating, they must also actually communicate. Where understanding by the patient is inevitably or demonstrably low, a particular duty of care arises, especially if there is potential harm. Team work, colleagues' advice or even the courts may need to be involved in the protection from risk of vulnerable individuals.

Doctors must be confident in their own skills at getting to the nub of a patient's problem as fully and accurately as possible. They must be aware of their limitations. Even within their own field with a skill that was once learned, there is a special duty of care if that skill has not been exercised recently or often. 'Having a go', whether at psychotherapy, surgery or syringing ears is indefensible, an issue relevant to nurses and others in health care considering expanding their roles. Making assumptions in history taking is indefensible. Leaving out the investigations which rule out the uncommon but serious is indefensible. It follows that doctors must always be self-aware and self-critical. They may also be self-satisfied if assessment of their work by themselves or by others shows that they are above the norm for good work in their field. What they may not be is complacent or set in their ways. They must be willing to refine and develop what they do, even what they do every day, as times and techniques change. 'The habits of a lifetime' may have become potentially harmful almost unnoticed in the hurly-burly of a busy professional life.

There is also an obligation on doctors to assess the potential risks of harm not only in their clinical practice but also in the physical surroundings, organisational set-up, financial circumstances, team arrangements and administrative support within which they work. These may be within their own capacity to adjust, especially in private practice or in NHS general practice, which they must then act upon. Where others provide the infrastructure, doctors should become involved in trying to ensure the elimination of potential patient harm. Blaming 'them' will not do if no action has been taken to tell 'them' about potentially harmful shortcomings. Doctors must ensure in all that they do that all known systems are in place and used to ensure the avoidance of common errors and of identified uncommon but potentially serious errors. They must assess the risks of new ideas or techniques and ensure that effective avoidance systems are created, put in place and are used and work.

Doctors must ensure that all equipment they use, including the basic content of consulting rooms, is fit for the purpose required, is properly maintained and renewed when necessary. They must know how to use the equipment properly and safely and must always do so.

Doctors must ensure that their own procedures for the preservation of patient confidentiality are complete and kept in such a way that confidential information is shared only on a need to know basis within systems that preserve confidentiality. Major harm to patients can result from breaches of confidence (MDU, 2001). Professional rules are clear but modern communication and data retention systems, and the legislation going with them, have concentrated and complicated this duty. The UK NHS is in the early stages of developing a universal electronic health record. This has clear clinical benefits but poses problems of confidentiality, identification and access.

Doctors have an obligation to communicate clearly with colleagues who are also involved, or to be involved, in the care of a particular patient. Record keeping must be clear, complete, concise, accurate, legible, relevant and timely. The records must be available when required – often a major administrative task – but securely held. Where patient care is shared, communication is even more important, especially in acute circumstances or in complex ongoing situations. Handover arrangements must be clear and comprehensive and must be used if patient harm through inadequate information is to be avoided.

Doctors must accept personal responsibility for what they personally do, or decide not to do. If they have told a patient that they will do or arrange something they must do so. Organisational sloppiness can cause patient harm, especially if it results in delay.

Doctors must ensure that they have time for themselves, not just to catch up with written work or reading, but to protect themselves as individuals, share life with their nearest and dearest, and sustain their self-worth and self-esteem outside the work environment. The work-obsessed diminish themselves and those around them and cannot bring to their patient interactions the open, observant mind which is the key to avoiding patient harm.

Doctors must recognise when they need a holiday. They should be self-aware enough to know when they are becoming over-whelmed, burned out, depressed, anxious, over fond of a drink or tempted to misuse the drugs to which they have easy access. They should have the courage to admit these problems and seek help. When they are ill, mentally or physically, they should seek advice in the same way as everyone else and not buttonhole a colleague in the corridor, or self-diagnose and self-medicate. The buttonholed should give the good advice that help should be sought elsewhere through appropriate routes. Doctors should give in when they must, so avoiding patient harm, and not wait for disciplinary or registration bodies to make them give in. There should be recog-nition of the duty to advise, warn and help colleagues with pro-blems. There should be a willingness to 'whistle blow' where appropriate, not only on personal or health grounds, but also on grounds of identifiable poor standards.

Doctors should listen fully, carefully and properly to their patients and be open to observation, including adverse comment and criticism. Explanations should be clear, failure acknowledged and good suggestions for change acted on. The customer is not always right, but should always understand what it is intended should happen, what has happened, and why. Openness greatly diminishes the potential for patient harm.

## Conclusion

All of the above principles are relevant to nurses and all other health professionals taking on wider autonomous roles which increasingly involve acting on personal judgements derived from personal skills in obtaining all relevant information from and about the patient. Knowing that such judgements will occasionally be wrong, no matter how carefully arrived at, and living with that knowledge, is part of the professionalism which greater autonomy requires and gives.

Elimination of all risk and harm in medical care is not possible. Inevitable or unavoidable risk can be minimised by good training and lifelong support for doctors and other health care professionals. Patients can reduce harm to themselves by always reporting promptly when things do not seem to be going as expected. To do that they must know clearly what is expected. Recognising and removing failing or misplaced individuals from the front line of patient care can avoid indefensible harm. A state run health care delivery system must set a corporate ethos dedicated to enabling the health care professionals to do their job properly by providing an infrastructure within which everyone else does their job properly as well.

Avoidance of harm to patients is thus much more than doctors simply doing the correct thing in the correct way for the individual patient. Doctors have a wider duty to other patients, to and for colleagues, to the organisation and infrastructure within which they work and to society as a whole, in order to build and sustain a professional life dedicated to 'first, do no harm.'

On December 6, 1617 King James I of England granted a Royal Charter to the Worshipful Society of Apothecaries of London, a guild of the city. He said 'These men have art as well as mysterie'. He meant that they could be relied upon to practice well and properly. Today's society expects the same.

## References

BMJ (1993) *Rationing in action*. BMJ Publishing Group, London.

CHI (2001) *Investigation into Loughborough GP*. Commission for Health Improvement, London.

DoH (1998a) *Our Healthier Nation*. Department of Health, London.

DoH (1998b) *The New NHS*. Department of Health, London.

DoH (2000a) *Supporting Doctors, Protecting Patients*. Chief Medical Officer of England, Department of Health, London.

DoH (2000b) *An Organisation with a Memory. Report of an expert group on learning from adverse events in the NHS, chaired by the Chief Medical Officer*. Department of Health, London.

DoH (2001) *Building a Safer NHS for Patients: Implementing 'An Organisation with a Memory'*. Department of Health, London.

Ford, J. (2001) *Apothecary 2001*. The Worshipful Society of Apothecaries, London.

GMC (1997) *Fitness to Practise Procedures*. General Medical Council of the UK, London.

GMC (2001a) *Tomorrow's Doctors – consultation document*. General Medical Council of the UK, London.

GMC (2001b) *Good Medical Practice*. General Medical Council of the UK, London.

Health Departments of the United Kingdom (1998) *First Report of the National Screening Committee*. Department of Health, London.

Herbert, I. (2001) *The Independent*. 9 October 2001, *Review*, p. 9.

MDU (2000) *Significant Event Audit*. Medical Defence Union Risk Management Services, London.

MDU (2001) *Confidentiality*. Medical Defence Union Services Ltd, London.

NHS (2001a) *Modernising Regulation in the Health Professions – consultation document*. Department of Health, London.

NHS (2001b) *Assuring the Quality of Medical Practice.* National Health Service Publications, London, England.

NHS Executive (1999a) *The Public Interest Disclosure Act; Whistleblowing in the NHS.* Health Service Circular 1999/198, London.

NHS Executive (1999b) *Clinical Governance in the New NHS.* Health Service Circular 1999/065, London.

Porter, R. (1997) *The Greatest Benefit to Mankind.* Harper Collins, London.

Shaw, G. B. (1911) *The Doctor's Dilemma.* Penguin, London.

Taylor, S. (Lord Taylor of Harlow) (1954) *Good General Practice.* Oxford University Press, London.

Williamson, C. (1992) *Whose Standards?* Open University Press, Buckingham.

van Zwanenberg, T. & Harrison, J. (eds) (2000) *Clinical Governance in Primary Care.* Radcliffe Medical Press, Abingdon.

# 13. *Limiting Harm in Future Health Care – The Role of Nursing*

*Frank Milligan and Kate Robinson*

'The unlucky learn from their mistakes. The lucky learn from others' mistakes'.

Sudanese camel herders' proverb (allegedly)

## Introduction

In this book, we have focused on the harm that can occur within our health care system. This is obviously a somewhat limited perspective in as much as it tends to neglect the vast amount of positive work that is undertaken by practitioners within the NHS and private health sectors. Of course it is the case that the majority of people working within the health systems of the UK are highly motivated and diligent. But doing good work and being highly motivated does not preclude any individual from causing harm. Although some of the text in the book has focused on individuals with malign intentions, such as Harold Shipman, the important messages are for all of us – those practitioners whose intentions are entirely honourable but who may cause harm to patients which can be prevented. For a range of reasons, and some of these have been described in this book, the limitations of current systems and the harm perpetuated within the NHS seem to be becoming clear. This harm ranges from the 25,000 estimated annual preventable deaths from adverse events in the NHS (Bristol Royal Infirmary Inquiry, 2001), to the problems inherent in children being labelled hyperactive (Chapter 6). These two very different examples help to illustrate the diverse nature of the unnecessary harm addressed here – and its complex motivation. This final chapter reflects briefly on some of the evidence presented and looks at possible strategies by which unnecessary harm might be reduced, and particularly at the potential roles for nurses in this endeavour. It is not intended to be a description of government policy on these issues, not least because we believe that reducing the harm done by the health care system will require action by a range of interested parties including individuals, NHS organisations, lay organisations and professional bodies, as well as the government. In a pluralistic society, the government does not control all the relevant levers for change, and practitioners also have the power to influence events.

## *Current UK government initiatives*

When the Labour party came to power in 1997 they placed a fundamental emphasis on improving quality in the NHS. The most visible manifestation of this policy was the explicit establishment of clinical governance (NHS Executive, 1999). It could be argued that the government were surprised by the paucity of channels through which they could affect the outcomes of care provided through the NHS. Previously, all the focus had been on the achievement of financial targets – clinical performance had been seen as a 'black box' which nobody knew anything about. This assumption changed with the publication of the White Paper, *The NHS, Modern and Dependable* (NHS Executive, 1997) that set out the reasons why assessing and managing performance in the NHS needed to change. This publication was quickly followed by *A First Class Service: Quality in the new NHS* (DoH, 1998), which clarified the means through which this quality agenda would be implemented.

So the first part of the policy framework which brought the actual provision of care to centre stage was the establishment of clinical governance. This was an essentially local framework of procedures and processes through which clinical care might be improved, and managers might know about the clinical standards of their organisation – for which they were, for the first time, accountable. This local framework was potentially supportive of the notion of individual practitioners developing evidence based practice. However, this left the question of local variation outstanding, as well as the reasonable assumption that senior figures in the research and policy communities could assess the data better than local practitioners. The government therefore established processes and organisations for setting national standards. These included National Service Frameworks (NSFs) related to different areas of care and the National Institute for Clinical Excellence (NICE). The NSFs spell out the evidence base of how services can be best organised for patients with particular health problems to those working in health care (there is, for example, a NSF for coronary heart disease). The NICE supplements this by providing guidance on clinical and cost effectiveness, for example through the assessment of drugs, devices and new treatments. An example of this can be found in Chapter 6 which explores the use of methylphenidate in children. Clinical governance is therefore a process through which each part of the NHS quality assures its clinical decisions. Other key elements of clinical governance include increased patient/public involvement and changes to professional regulation and education. The degree to which national standards were being maintained was to be monitored by the Commission for Health Improvement (CHI), soon to become the Commission for Healthcare Audit and Inspection (CHAI), a national performance framework and patient/user surveys (DoH, 1998).

There was little mention of harm or adverse events at this stage of the government's agenda – whether the scale of the problem was unknown or there was a reluctance to act is unclear. However, the problem was addressed through the publication of the document *An Organisation with a Memory* (DoH, 2000). This marked a significant shift in the focus on harm reduction within UK health care and added a new dimension to the clinical governance agenda. This document was a comprehensive report by an expert group charged with identifying the means by which adverse events could be more clearly identified and the lessons learnt. Essentially the document was an open admission of the scale and extent of the problem – that too many preventable adverse health care events occur in the NHS. Furthermore, it acknowledged that some of the errors made have been repeated over a number of years. It is claimed in the opening of the document that such events are uncommon when compared with the volume of work undertaken within the NHS, but this does not correspond with the evidence cited here in Chapter 2 (see, for example, Brennan *et al.*, 1991; Leape *et al.*, 1991; Wilson *et al.*, 1995; Leape, 1999; Vincent *et al.*, 2001) which suggests that they are not uncommon enough. The Department of Health followed the report with a second publication, *Building a Safer NHS for Patients* (DoH, 2001b) that outlined how *An Organisation with a Memory*, and therefore harm reduction, would be implemented.

Adverse events are defined as '... an event or omission arising during clinical care and causing physical or psychological injury to a patient' (DoH, 2000 p. xii). It is acknowledged in the report that not only do adverse events lead to distress and death, but also that they cost the NHS about £400 million a year in the settlement of clinical negligence claims. The report also acknowledges that current research, and this includes that mentioned in the last paragraph, does not give an accurate indication of the real size of the problem. In other words, it acknowledges that the problem of adverse events is probably more widespread than current research indicates. The recommendations made within the document were to:

i.    introduce a mandatory reporting scheme for adverse events and specified near misses
ii.   introduce a scheme for confidential reporting by staff of adverse events and near misses
iii.  encourage a reporting and questioning culture in the NHS
iv.   introduce a single overall system for analysing and disseminating lessons from adverse events and near misses
v.    make better use of existing sources of information on adverse events
vi.   improve the quality and relevance of NHS adverse event investigations and inquiries
vii.  undertake a programme of basic research into adverse events in the NHS
viii. make full use of new NHS information systems to help staff access learning from adverse health care events
ix.   act to ensure that important lessons are implemented quickly and consistently
x.    identify and address specific categories of serious recurring adverse health care events.

These recommendations gave a clear signal to nurses and other practitioners in health care that the government takes harm reduction seriously and intends to deal with it on both a local and national basis.

   The following year, the consultation document entitled *Doing Less Harm* (DoH, 2001a) took the harm reduction initiative one step further and set out key requirements for local organisations to manage, report, analyse and learn from adverse events. It suggested that awareness and understanding of adverse events must be improved along with systems to manage and report these locally. There should also be a fast-track process for serious incidents, which will be called 'category red'. This category includes a near miss that would have seriously harmed the patient and/or the organisation. The document makes it clear that the guidance is intended to apply to all individuals involved either directly or indirectly in patient care. An adverse patient incident is defined as:

> '... any event or circumstance arising during NHS care that could have or did lead to unintended or unexpected harm, loss or damage. Harm is injury (physical or psychological), disease, suffering, disability or death.'
>
> DoH, 2001a p. 13

It is acknowledged that some such events are already well known, for example surgical complications, but local organisations will be charged with providing suitable guidance on reporting and monitoring such incidents. Many of the examples of unnecessary harm identified within this book fit this description and that of an 'adverse event' as defined above (DoH, 2000). Further details on the structures and mechanisms involved were clarified in *Building a Safer NHS for Patients* (DoH, 2001b) and the response to the Bristol Royal Infirmary Inquiry (DoH, 2002).

A key body that has been established within the national clinical governance framework is the National Patient Safety Agency. Its remit is to coordinate efforts to report and learn from adverse events occurring in the NHS (NPSA, 2002) and its core purpose is: '... to improve patient safety by reducing risk of harm through error' (DoH, 2001b p. 4). It will work closely with other established bodies in the NHS, including the Commission for Health Improvement (CHI) and NICE, adding yet another dimension to the quality agenda in the NHS. Leape (1999), in an analysis of error in medicine that drew parallels with developments in aviation, noted that one of the significant advances in aviation safety in the USA was the creation of independent agencies that set safety standards to which the airline industry is required to adhere. The claimed independence of the patient safety agency (NPSA, 2002) is to be welcomed, although quite how independent it will be remains to be seen.

Another area of development is that related to patient involvement and patient advocacy. Chapter 8 described the systems previously operating in the NHS in support of patients who had problems and wished to make a complaint. At the time of writing (late 2002) the current local organisational framework for involving and supporting patients who have such problems is unclear, and this may be in part because of the difficulties of incorporating patients into formal structures while maintaining their independence. We are currently looking at the formation of Patient Advice and Liaison Services (PALSs), which are part of the planned replacement for the Community Health Councils (see Chapter 8). These will operate locally to provide a network through which patients and their carers can be supported thus ensuring that concerns about NHS services are identified early and dealt with. The Department of Health wants a PALS in every NHS Primary Care Trust in England to resolve problems on the spot before they become more serious (DoH, 2002). This is part of the patient empowerment agenda which also seeks to involve local government more closely in local service provision.

It is therefore clear that significant change is taking place – change that involves elements of central and local government bureaucracy and incorporates more lay public involvement and scrutiny of the work of the NHS. Before moving on to the incidence and cost of clinical negligence, it is important to acknowledge that the push to improve quality has embraced the everyday aspects of nursing care. The document *The Essence of Care* (DoH, 2001e), which again has its roots in the clinical governance agenda (NHS Executive, 1998), explores and encourages the use of benchmarks to improve the quality of fundamental aspects of care and contains tools to help practitioners achieve this. It is acknowledged that it is the 'softer aspects of care', such as maintaining patients' privacy and dignity, that are crucial to quality and that these should, therefore, be the subject of scrutiny and benchmarking.

## Clinical negligence and compensation

The motivators for the changes outlined above include a variety of reasons described elsewhere in this book, but a highly significant factor is the increasing costs faced through adverse events that lead to litigation. As already noted, the NHS pays out an estimated £400 million a year in clinical negligence claims and adverse events cost around £2 billion a year in additional hospital stays (DoH, 2001b). Furthermore, the provision for clinical negligence liability is estimated to have increased by £500 million in 2000/01 to a figure of £4.4 billion (Mayor, 2002). Although the Department of Heath accepted many of the findings of the Bristol Royal Infirmary Inquiry, it was uncertain about the recommendation that clinical negligence claims should be abolished (DoH, 2002). The DoH (2001c) has, however, noted that the current system is bureaucratic and slow. Cases completed in 1999/00 took an average of five and a half years to close with legal costs often exceeding the payments which claimants receive.

The NHS Litigation Authority was set up in April 2000 and

assumed responsibility for the administration of all negligence cases (Mayor, 2002). This move, along with collaboration between other governmental departments under the *Co-ordination of Reviews of Risk Management in NHS Bodies in England and Wales* (NHS Reviews Co-ordination Group, 2002), demonstrates that strategic attempts are being made to enhance understanding of adverse events, especially those that are claimed as negligence. This mechanism will also facilitate the centralisation of data collection on those adverse events that lead to negligence claims. There was also some duplication of the audit of Trust work by the bodies that form the Co-ordination Group, for example in evaluating complaints procedures. This duplication should now be reduced, thereby cutting the workload of the governmental agencies as well as the Trusts which had to provide the information.

## Limiting medical harm in health care

The initiatives and changes to the NHS described in outline above are clearly aimed at improving quality in the NHS, and a significant reduction in the incidence of adverse events is central to that goal. The work of Sharpe and Faden (1998) is now explored to give another, in many ways complementary, view of harm reduction. Sharpe and Faden are a rare example of authors prepared to offer clear suggestions on strategies for limiting medical harm. In the conclusion of their book on the subject they suggest the following as strategies central to harm reduction: surveillance; information technology; systems analysis; education (overcoming the ethos of infallibility in medical education), and, finally, expanding the evidentiary basis of practice. These are now explored, in the order given by Sharpe and Faden, and limits to the critique they offer highlighted. Where appropriate, links with earlier chapters and current initiatives are made.

### Surveillance strategies

Surveillance has been a recurrent theme throughout this book. Surveillance within health care can operate on a number of levels. These range from the surveillance of systems to ensure that they are functioning efficiently through to monitoring of the individual health care staff and patients. In this latter sense surveillance can constitute a form of social iatrogenesis as described in Chapter 2: aspects of people's lives become increasingly subject to the gaze, the concern and work, of health care practitioners.

Adverse drug reactions are given as an example by Sharpe and

Faden of where active surveillance has brought positive benefits in health care. They argue that active surveillance has identified a dramatically higher incidence of adverse drug reactions than are reported in traditional passive systems. In the latter, problems are only reported after they have occurred. A shift to more active surveillance rests on the assumption that problems will occur, and research has shown that medical staff tend not to operate from such a perspective (Leape, 1999; Sexton *et al.*, 2000). The yellow card scheme for reporting adverse drug reactions in England, Scotland and Wales is claimed to be one of the best in the world, but there is still a degree of under-reporting (DoH, 2001a). The Department of Health are instigating mandatory reporting for adverse health care events and specified near misses which may help to identify drug related problems, although this remains by nature, a passive system. The Department of Health target is to reduce by 40% the number of serious errors in the use of prescribed drugs by 2005 (DoH, 2001b). Furthermore, drug prescription and administration systems are in need of revision within the NHS and private sectors, where there remains a reliance upon handwritten prescriptions. These are inevitably more difficult to monitor than electronic systems. There is of course no systematic reporting system for herbal remedies and the other substances mentioned in Chapter 5.

However, Sharpe and Faden do not make clear reference to the possible rise in, and potential value of, surveillance of individual practitioners. Recent adverse publicity on the medical profession in the UK, for example the cases of Shipman (Baker, 2001; Smith, 2002) and Ledward (Ritchie Report, 2000) (general practitioner and gynaecologist respectively) and the Bristol Royal Infirmary Inquiry (2001; DoH, 2002) have helped to create a perception that more surveillance of individual medical practitioners is required. The UK government put forward proposals to deal with poor clinical performance in *Supporting Doctors, Protecting Patients* document (DoH, 1999) and intensified the debate around current error levels in health care through the report on adverse events in the NHS (DoH, 2000; 2001b). Again, these initiatives appear central to harm reduction and should be the concern of nursing staff in terms of seeing them initiated and maintained. Although an increase in surveillance brings with it a sense of loss with regard to personal liberty, it seems inevitable that it will occur in the attempt to reduce unnecessary harm through ill judged and occasionally malicious practice. It is likely that the surveillance of other health care staff will increase – and the example of surveillance within the NHS Direct system has been given here (Chapter 11). As is common in many telephone call centres, calls can be recorded and within the NHS Direct system such recordings are subsequently used to monitor and evaluate the performance of nursing staff.

## Information technology

Although so much of our everyday lives are influenced and supported by IT in its various guises, there arguably remains within modern health care an over-reliance on human judgement, a position that mirrors medical faith in the rational decision making of its individual practitioners (see Chapter 12). Nevertheless, health care is complex and, as the literature on error reduction has shown, human judgement alone is notoriously unreliable (Leape, 1999). With this in mind the significance of the NHS Direct initiative described in Chapter 11 should not be underestimated. There is evidence that doctors have been reluctant to use computer technology to support the assessment and diagnostic element of their work. For example, experimental work in computer-aided diagnosis was undertaken between 1969 and 1983 on around 30,000 cases of abdominal pain in the UK. This showed that such methods could significantly increase the rate of accurate diagnosis (de Dombal, 1991). However, such early developments have not been adopted on a wider scale. In contrast, medicine has been keen to use computer technology to enhance its gaze of the biological body and a plethora of imaging and screening devices are now found in hospitals. Following the precedent of NHS Direct, it seems likely that computerised algorithms will become more common in clinical practice supporting the assessment of a range of health care problems.

Similarly, much of health care in the UK remains reliant upon handwritten notes and prescriptions even though these inevitably lead to poor communication, problems with the continuity of care, and a multitude of errors. It would be inappropriate to criticise the practitioners too strongly on this matter, especially as the development and purchase of such systems lies, in part at least, outside their remit, but significant health improvements appear achievable through expanding the use of IT for these purposes (Bristol Royal Infirmary Inquiry, 2001; DoH, 2002). As mentioned above, many drug prescriptions in UK hospitals are still handwritten and not verified through computerised systems that check dosage, potential drug interactions and even cross-reference with various patient test results and diagnostic categories. Bates (2000) argues that there is a great deal of benefit to be gained through the use of such technology. He cites evidence that between 28% and 56% of adverse drug events are preventable. A range of evidence on this matter was reviewed in Chapter 5. Systems already exist to match patients to their drug chart, reducing the risk of them receiving the wrong (often another patient's) drugs, a problem with which many nurses are familiar.

The potential need for increasing use of IT in the ward arena has been supported by recent research by Neale *et al.* (2001), extending the work of Vincent *et al.* (2001). This sought to quantify the number of adverse events that occur in British hospitals (see Chapter 2), and found that 53% of the adverse events identified occurred in general ward care. The study involved a review of 1,014 records from two different hospital sites. The category of general ward care included aspects such as patient assessment, pressure sore prevention, and the use of drugs and intravenous fluids. Although it was only a pilot study, albeit one based upon widely accepted research methods in this area (see for example Brennan *et al.*, 1991; Leape *et al.*, 1991; Wilson *et al.*, 1995), the work suggests that the majority of adverse events are linked to the ward environment. In the UK, at this time, this is an environment that contains little in the way of information technology to aid patient assessment, diagnosis, care planning, drug prescription and administration. Sharpe and Faden (1998) also argued that electronic medical records (health records may be a better term), will enhance communication between practitioners and reduce duplication and error. In the UK, the government has identified a range of goals in relation to information technology (NHS Executive, 1998; DoH, 2001b). They include the introduction of lifelong electronic records and round the clock online access to patient records as well as information about best clinical practice by the year 2005. The division between notes held by GPs and hospital records will be broken. This change alone may significantly improve communication and continuity and reduce the need to duplicate some clinical tests.

As with any innovation, the increasing use of IT brings with it potential disadvantages. Some critics (see Chapters 8 and 12) are concerned about the possible reduction in face to face contact between health practitioners and the patient/client. Other concerns include the threat to confidentiality and what happens when these systems go wrong. Discussion with regard to the former ought to include the concept of surveillance. The ability of health care practitioners and others working in the public and private sectors, both in and outside of health care, to monitor the behaviour and movements of the public is powerfully enhanced through the use of IT. Even so, it is difficult to envisage anything other than significant changes in health care in terms of the utilisation of IT. On balance, and after taking into consideration the potential problems described above, information technology seems to have much to offer health care practitioners in terms of reducing harm, a position supported by the Bristol Royal Infirmary Inquiry (2001) and the official response to it (DoH, 2002).

## Systems analysis

In terms of systems analysis, Sharpe and Faden (1989) suggest that organisations avoid the 'bad apple' approach of blaming individuals when errors occur. This has been accepted by the UK government (DoH, 2000; 2001b; 2002), although such a shift in culture will no doubt prove difficult to encourage within the NHS. Through comprehensive systems analysis, a more accurate picture of the contributory reasons for an adverse incident can be gained. The Department of Health (DoH, 2000; 2001b) describe a systems approach as a holistic stance on the issue of failure, one that embraces multiple aspects of the organisation including people, teams, tasks, workplaces and institutions. An essential challenge within this will be to facilitate a situation in which medical staff see themselves as simply part of the team, and not necessarily the leader or key member. These issues were discussed in Chapters 2, 4 and 9 in the context of nurses working with medical staff within a culture that reflects a historical subservience to the medical profession. Within such an environment nursing staff can find it difficult to express their concerns, a problem described in the doctor–nurse game (Stein, 1967; Stein *et al.*, 1990) and as found in empirical research that traces the cause of errors in clinical practice (for example Boreham *et al.*, 2000). The deference sometimes expected by medicine, or perceived to be appropriate by other health care staff, almost certainly contributes to adverse events occurring (Boreham *et al.*, 2000; DoH, 2002).

Leape (1999) has explored the high error rates in medicine and compared its limited approach to error reduction with research from other fields, notably aviation. One of the key differences between aviation and medicine is that the former assumes that errors will occur, and that people will make mistakes. This is generally not the case in medicine and this attitude can be seen within the systems currently operating within much of UK health care. The central point being made by Leape (1999) and others is that error reduction has to embrace human, technological and systems factors. One of the problems has been that medicine, as a profession, frequently appears to see itself as being above such scrutiny.

Evidence for this claim can be found in the work of Sexton *et al.* (2000). They conducted a large international survey comparing the attitudes of operating theatre and intensive care unit staff with those of airline cockpit crew. The outcome measures obtained related to perceptions of error, stress and teamwork. They found that pilots were the least likely to deny the effects of fatigue on performance (26% compared with 70% of surgeons and 47% of anaesthetists) and consultant surgeons were the least likely to advocate flat hierarchies. In other words, they were the least likely to take advice from junior members of staff, be they medical or non-medical. The impression gained from the Sexton study is that pilots were generally prepared to acknowledge their limitations and listen to others from lower down the hierarchy, whereas consultant surgeons were much more reluctant to do so. The problem is neatly summarised thus: 'In aviation, perceptions of fatigue and stress, and error continue to be topics of training and targets for improvements', and further, 'We found that susceptibility to error is not universally acknowledged by medical staff, and many report that error is not handled appropriately in their hospital' (Sexton *et al.*, 2000 p. 747). This point brings into focus the challenge faced in trying to generate a blame free culture (Sharpe & Faden, 1998; DoH, 2000).

Although aviation seems somewhat distant and different from health care, research and debate from that field on error reduction is widely accepted as being of relevance (see for example Leape, 1999; DoH, 2002). As described above in the section on current government initiatives, there are significant changes in place and planned within the NHS to improve the focus upon adverse events. It is clear that a systems approach is central to this and that lessons from aviation, such as the promotion of a blame free culture and the formation of independent bodies to oversee professional groups is part of this (DoH, 2000, 2002). The system will include increased patient/public involvement, for example through the Patient Advice Liaison Services (PALSs), through to enhanced coordination and cooperation between various governmental bodies charged with managing aspects of health care and reducing risk (DoH, 2001d; 2002; National Health Service Reviews Co-ordination Group, 2002).

## Educational changes

One of the most controversial suggestions Sharpe and Faden (1998) make is that the ethos of infallibility inherent in medical education needs to be addressed. As described above, the socialisation of doctors has tended to emphasise perfectibility and infallibility. There has been a lack of focus on error prevention, and where considered there has been an emphasis on specific incidents and individuals rather than systems failures. This ethos of infallibility is reinforced by the assumption that scientific knowledge generates objective truth and that deference should be given to authorities that display such knowledge. The interesting point here is that philosophers such as Popper have successfully argued that reductionist science often makes progress through error and correction, and so fallibility is a necessary component of intellectual growth. For these reasons McIntyre and Popper (1983) called for the systematic recording of all medical errors. This approach, they argue, would not condemn or denigrate practitioners but educate and improve performance.

This is a far from new idea and can be traced back to the work of Ernest Codman (1869–1940), circa 1913 (Sharpe & Faden, 1998). Codman, a physician in Boston, Massachusetts, offered the 'end result' system in which a hospital would follow through each patient it treated to determine if the treatment was successful or not. If it was not, then the hospital was charged with finding out 'why not'? The pressures to expand clinical audit (DoH, 2002) may perhaps see some of Codman's efforts acknowledged. Although clinical audit, which in itself is a form of surveillance, offers a strategy through which clinicians receive feedback on their performance and harmful practice can, it is hoped, be detected early, the efficacy of such programmes remains debatable. What will happen to the results of such audit and how will clinicians, and those charged with management of the organisations, respond to them. Ironically Rodney Ledward (Ritchie Report, 2000) introduced clinical audit into the NHS hospital in which he worked, but it neither operated effectively nor picked up the vagaries of his practice. Audit conducted within any profession by members of that profession runs the risk of being short of objectivity, a notion supported by some within medicine itself (Sellwood, 2000).

Parallels can be drawn between the Department of Health's response to the Bristol Royal Infirmary Inquiry (DoH, 2002), Codman's work and the claims of McIntyre and Popper (1983). The Department of Health's response called for publication of 30 day mortality rates for every cardiac surgeon in England, along with other published data on clinical performance for consultants, their units and teams. It seems clear then that clinical performance within the NHS will be subject to increased surveillance and reporting. Quite how this will affect the private sector remains to be seen.

These, and other initiatives mentioned in this final chapter, offer significant challenges for those planning and providing both medical and nurse education.

## Evidence based practice

There have been substantial efforts made within health care in the UK to raise the evidence base of practice. Comments put forward by Sharpe and Faden (1998) on the state of evidentiary practice in medicine appear highly relevant to nursing as well. They argue that evidence tends to emphasise efficiency as opposed to effectiveness. The former refers to the level of benefit achieved under ideal conditions whereas effectiveness is the response gained in 'normal' treatment conditions. They also argue that physicians can lack the skills to interpret and utilise such evidence effectively. Nursing and other health care disciplines in the UK, such as physiotherapy and occupational therapy, have raised their academic standards in recent times and this may help them to evaluate and to implement research findings more effectively. However, what Sharpe and Faden do not acknowledge in relation to expanding the evidentiary basis of medicine is the potentially limited nature of the evidence itself. Within medical discourse, certain forms of evidence will invariably carry more weight. Examples of this were given in several of the earlier chapters: the drift towards drug therapy for children displaying disruptive behaviour; the priority given to biomedical interventions in some aspects of mental health practice; and the medicalisation of the dying process. Aspects of health care associated with intervention and technology may therefore take priority and the evaluation of health related evidence should be undertaken with this in mind. It is worth making one last point in relation to evidence based practice – that some innovations proceed despite a lack of evidence. NHS Direct is an example of this but one supported through many of the arguments given in this book.

## Reducing harm: the role of nursing

We have suggested that nursing is now operating in a managerial context which supports the school of thought that proper consideration is given to the ways in which unnecessary harm and adverse events can be reduced (DoH, 2001b; 2002) and, indeed, increasingly requires it. The areas described above by Sharpe and Faden (1998) provide the beginnings of a coherent strategy to reduce harm in health care in general, although they were directed at medicine. The work of Neale *et al.* (2001) should particularly raise concerns for many nursing staff, as it suggests that the hospital ward, one of the key areas for delivering nursing care, can be a dangerous place for patients. Although there has been little direct reference to the general ward within this book, there is increasing evidence that the environment, and the work that takes place within it, is potentially harmful in a number of ways. The Neale *et al.* study included aspects of care that directly relate to nursing responsibilities, for example pressure sore prevention and discharge planning. In addition, we know that hospital acquired infections kill around 5,000 people a year in the UK (Comptroller and Auditor General, 2000) and that the nutritional support that people receive whilst hospitalised is generally poor (Burke, 1997). And, although nursing care increasingly takes place outside of the ward we should not assume that other areas do not carry equivalent risks. Clearly there is a considerable agenda of research waiting to be done.

Although Chapter 3 highlighted a problem with professionalisation, it could be argued that the adoption of a 'proper' professional attitude will help nurses tackle the challenges described and analysed in this book. Davies (1995, p. 135) distinguishes

'... between a broad sense of professionalism as probity or integrity of personal conduct and professionalism/professionalization as a route taken collectively by members of an occupational group who refine and guard their knowledge base, set boundaries around who can enter and what the limits of practice will be...'.

It is the former, rather than the latter, which should underpin the culture change required.

## Conclusion

This book has brought together a range of diverse evidence demonstrating first, that health care systems dominated by western medicine may themselves cause unnecessary harm, and second, that governments, patients and practitioners alike are beginning to address these issues. We have also been concerned to address the issue that the nature and extent of this harm remains largely hidden, although both medicine and health care generally face increasing challenges from a more informed public and a rising critique of the professional project. The concept of iatrogenic harm has been shown to help identify and quantify the extent of the problems faced by those working in health care. It has also been suggested that, because nursing is a discipline closely allied to medicine, it can find it difficult to evaluate the limitations of western medicine objectively in relation to health care in its broadest sense. This may be an increasingly important issue as nursing finds itself taking on aspects of medical work, the work practices of which are based upon assumptions which are themselves limited. The historically close relationship which nursing has with medicine, and the status advantage held by the latter, contributes to a perspective that lacks a clear focus on what is commonly claimed as the goal of nursing – health. If nursing is truly interested in promoting health then factors that have a negative impact on it are worthy of scrutiny. The evidence cited in this book suggests that modern health care, health care that has been heavily influenced by western medicine, is worthy of such scrutiny, as are all those that work within the systems used therein. Perhaps the most important step towards reducing iatrogenic harm is to put it on the map and to value it as a concept relevant to the effective planning and delivery of health care. The reference to maps in Chapter 1 was an attempt to introduce the type of thinking that will be required. The recent government initiatives to reduce adverse health care events provide a welcome lead and clear guidance on ways in which this can be done (DoH, 2000; 2001a; 2001b; 2002).

In conclusion, the British comedian Peter Cook, playing the part of a retired army officer in a sketch with Dudley Moore, was asked if he had learnt from his mistakes. He replied, 'Of course I have, and I could repeat them all again exactly!' This rather ironically sums up the problems of the NHS as described in the recent document *An Organisation with a Memory* (DoH, 2000). One of the clear messages behind that document was that those working in the NHS had not learnt from mistakes, even those involving loss of life. However, the harm described in this book through the examples and evidence cited has been about more than mistakes – it has been about culture. Just as the Peter Cook sketch was a comment on the patriarchal culture of the armed forces, the arrogance and intransigence that at times led to disasters, so this book reflects upon a medically influenced culture which has insufficiently valued external criticism and self-reflection. It is now appropriate and necessary to change this culture. We hope this book has contributed constructively towards such a critique.

# References

Baker, R. (2001) *Harold Shipman's Clinical Practice 1974–1998*. Department of Health, London.

Bates, D. W. (2000) Using information technology to reduce rates of medication errors in hospitals. *British Medical Journal*. **32**, 788–791.

Boreham, N. C., Shea, C. E. & Mackway-Jones K. (2000) Clinical risk in the hospital emergency department in the UK. *Social Science and Medicine*. **51**, 83–91.

Brennan, T. A., Leape, L. L., Laird, N. M., Hebert, L., Localio, A. R., Lawthers, A. G., Newhouse, J. P., Weiler, P. C. & Hiatt, H. H. (1991) Incidence of adverse events and negligence in hospitalized patients. Results of the Harvard Medical Practice Study I. *New England Journal of Medicine*. **324**, 370–376.

Bristol Royal Infirmary Inquiry (2001) *Learning from Bristol. The report of the public inquiry into children's heart surgery at the Bristol Royal Infirmary, 1984–1995*. Department of Health, London.

Burke, A. (1997) *Hungry in Hospital?* Association of Community Health Councils for England and Wales, London.

Comptroller and Auditor General (2000) *The Management and Control of Hospital Acquired Infection in Acute NHS Trusts in England*. Department of Health, London.

Davies, C. (1995) *Gender and the Professional Predicament in Nursing*. Open University Press, Buckingham.

de Dombal, F. T. (1991) Computer-aided diagnosis of acute abdominal pain: the British experience. In: *Professional Judgement: A reader in clinical decision making* (eds by J. Downie & A. Elstein), pp. 190–199. Cambridge University Press, Cambridge.

DoH (1998) *A First Class Service: Quality in the new NHS*. Department of Health, London.

DoH (1999) *Supporting Doctors, Protecting Patients*. DoH, London.

Department of Health (2000) *An Organisation with a Memory. Report of an expert group on learning from adverse events in the NHS chaired by the Chief Medical Officer*. The Stationery Office, London.

DoH (2001a) *Doing Less Harm. Improving the safety and quality of care through reporting, analysing and learning from adverse incidents involving NHS patients – key requirements for health care providers*. Consultation document. Department of Health & National Patient Safety Agency, London.

DoH (2001b) *Building a Safer NHS for Patients: Implementing 'An Organisation with a Memory'*. The Stationery Office and Department of Health, London.

DoH (2001c) *New clinical compensation scheme for the NHS*. Press Release 2002/0313. Department of Health, London.

DoH (2001d) *Involving Patients and the Public in Health Care: Response to the listening exercise*. Department of Health, London.

DoH (2001e) *The Essence of Care: Patient-focused benchmarking for health care practitioners*. The Stationery Office, London.

DoH (2002) *Learning from Bristol: The Department of Health's response to the Report of the Public Inquiry into children's heart surgery at the Bristol Royal Infirmary 1984–1995*. The Stationery Office, London.

Leape, L. L., Brennan, T. A., Laird, N. M., Lawthers, A. G., Localio, A. R., Barnes, B. A., Herbert, L., Newhouse, J. P., Weiler, P. C. & Hiatt, H. H. (1991) The nature of adverse events in hopsitalized patients. Results of the Harvard Medical Practice study II. *New England Journal of Medicine*. **324**, 377–384.

Leape, L. (1999) Error in medicine. In: *Medical Mishaps: Pieces of the puzzle* (eds M. M. Rosenthal, L. Mulcahy & S. Lloyd-Bostock), pp. 20–38. Open University Press, Buckingham.

Mayor, S. (2002) NHS faces increase of £500m in clinical negligence liability. *British Medical Journal*. **324**, 997.

McIntyre, N. & Popper, K. (1983) The critical attitude in medicine: the need for a new ethics. *British Medical Journal*. **287**, 1919–1923.

National Health Service Reviews Co-ordination Group (2002) *Co-ordination of Reviews of Risk Management in NHS Bodies in England and Wales – Principles of agreement between review organisations*. NHS Reviews Co-ordination Group, London.

Neale, G., Woloshynowych, M. & Vincent, C. (2001) Exploring the causes of adverse events in NHS hospital practice. *Journal of the Royal Society of Medicine*. **94**, 322–330.

NHS Executive (1997) *The New NHS, Modern and Dependable. A national framework for assessing performance*. Department of Health, London.

NHS Executive (1998) *Information for Health*. NHS Executive, London.

NHS Executive (1999) *Clinical Governance: Quality in the new NHS*. Department of Health, London.

NPSA (2002) *National Patient Safety Agency NHS*. http://www.npsa.org.uk/

Ritchie Report (2000) *Report of the Inquiry into Quality and Practice Within the National Health Service Arising from the Actions of Rodney Ledward*. Department of Health, London.

Sellwood, W. G. (2000) Ramifications of Ledward case (letter). *British Medical Journal*. **321**, 446.

Sexton, J. B., Thomas, E. J. & Helmreich, R. L. (2000) Error, stress, and teamwork in medicine and aviation: cross sectional surveys. *British Medical Journal*. **320**, 745–749.

Smith, D. J. (2002) *The Shipman Inquiry: Independent public inquiry into the issues arising from the case of Harold Shipman*. Department of Health, London.

Stein, E. I. (1967) The doctor–nurse game. *Archives of General Psychiatry*. **16**, 699–703.

Stein, L. T., Watts, D. T. & Howell, T. (1990) The doctor–nurse game revisited. *Nursing Outlook*. **38**, 264–268.

Sharpe, V. A. & Faden, A. I. (1998) *Medical Harm: Historical, conceptual, ethical dimensions of iatrogenic illness.* Cambridge University Press, Cambridge.

Vincent, C., Neale, G. & Woloshynowych, M. (2001) Adverse events in British hospitals: preliminary retrospective record review. *British Medical Journal.* **322**, 517–519.

Wilson, R., Runciman, W. B., Gibberd, R. W., Harrison, B. T., Newby, L. & Hamilton, J. D. (1995) The quality in Australian health care study. *Medical Journal of Australia.* **163**, 458–471.

# *Index*